⌘

Hot and Cold Health

Handbook of Natural Medicine East and West

****

RICHARD G. HEFT
Acupuncture Physician

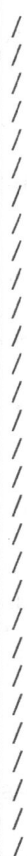

ISBN: 9780974791709
© 2003, Richard G. Heft
Revised 8/2025
R. G. Heft Publications
Email: richardgheft@aol.com

Disclaimer

All information contained herein is provided for general information purposes only and should not be considered as a substitute for medical consultation with a duly licensed health-care professional.

Special Thanks

1. Many authors I have read
2. **Michio Kushi**, **Aveline Kushi**, **Hamsa Newmark** and **Tonia Gagne** who taught me macrobiotic diet, how to cook natural foods tastefully, healthfully
3. **Customers** and **employees** from my health food store, Food and Thought, Hollywood, FL (1984- 2001) for their support, friendship
4. **Dan Nevel**, licensed Acupuncture Physician (L.Ac.) inspired me to study Traditional Chinese Medicine
5. **Dr. Richard Brown** OMD., **Nancy Brown**, CNC., owners, Acupressure Acupuncture Institute, Miami, FL
6. **Camillo Sanchez**, L.Ac., my first-year teacher
7. **Haley_graphics2** book cover designer @fiverr.com
8. **Lightning Source Inc.** printing, distribution, division of Ingram, independent author's best friend

TABLE OF CONTENTS

SUMMARY

Controlling energy (life-force of the body, all matter), elements (air, fire, water, earth) and nutrients (building, cleansing) via diet (animal, plant), herbs, exercise, sun, earth and spiritual practice is the science and combined natural healing practices of Naturopathy, Chinese Medicine and Ayurveda (India) that maintain health, normal structure, function, powers, pleasures, body, mind and spirit (Spirit), prevent and cure most disease, abnormal, weakness, pain. Everything changes. Nothing stays the same. Health, disease ⇨ better or worse.

BODY (health, disease) ⇨ created, preserved or destroyed by ENERGY via specific materials (elements, nutrients, poisons) and construction (thick, thin, watery, solid, hollow, etc.) ⇨ CHANGES daily ⇨ **better** (normal thick, thin, watery, strong, etc. structure function) or **worse** (abnormal, weak, too thick, thin, watery, deadly, etc.) ⇨ ongoing, predictable and mostly controllable product of **cause and effect**, <u>balance of opposites</u> ⇨
∧

1. Sun, earth, trees, plants, oxygen, carbon dioxide
2. Fruit, grain, sugar, dairy, chicken, coffee, herbs
3. Drugs, smoking, sex, exercise, pollution, etc. ⇨
- Create, build, fuel, heat, cool, expand, contract
- Move, hold, dry, air, moisten, thicken, thin
- Increase, decrease, purify or destroy
- Slowly, quickly, small to large ⇨

STRUCTURES: 30 trillion **cells** (30,000 billion) ⇨ billions (1,000 million) ⇨ specialized **tissues**: nerves (3 trillion), glands (7), organs (10), bones, muscles, skin; **vessels**: arteries, veins, capillaries (10 billion); hormones, blood, antibodies, lymph, mucus, acid, enzymes, urine ⇨ FUNCTIONS: vision, sleep, memory, respiration, digestion, circulation, cleansing, elimination, locomotion, immunity, reproduction **healthy**, **diseased**, stone, tumor, cancer ⇨ build-up, break down.

Most disease has **multiple** causes (#1- 3) and effects (symptoms), some that can be changed, eliminated; others not. Poor diet (varies) tends to dominate. Most diet-related disease, if not too severe, van be cured via **correct diet** and **herbs**, which is why myself (1- 4) and others I counseled (5- 7) or met (8) were able to cure:

1. Atherosclerosis, high blood pressure, angina
2. Arthritis, Restless Leg Syndrome, Plantar Fasciitis
3. Common cold, sore throat, insomnia, impotence
4. Obesity, poor vision, eczema, sour body odor
5. Neuralgia, GIRD, Irritable Bowel Syndrome, ADD
6. Anal fissure, psoriasis, edema, cellulite, sinusitis
7. Anemia, miscarriage, UTI, yeast infection, Crohn's
8. Diabetes mellitus, tumors, cancer (breast)

Correct diet (animal, plant, cooked, raw, etc.):

1. Varies: (a) many diseases have multiple dietary causes, poor diets (b) climate, (c) condition
- The same foods, herbs that help reverse, cure one disease, variation, may worsen another.

2. Centered: body's constitution, nutrient balance = 64% water, 16% protein (water-soluble), 16% fat, 4% minerals, <1% vitamins ⇨ **health** ⇨
- **Normal**: spongey, thick, thin, solid, watery, hollow, etc. tissues, vessels ⇨ expand, contract ⇨ continual movement, absorption, elimination, of blood, wastes, etc. in, out every tissue, cell.

3. Requires processing. Food, fluids ⇨
a) **Digestion** ⇨ stomach ⇨ *small* (24' tube) ⇨ *large intestine* (5') ⇨ acid, enzymes, bile, etc. ⇨ reduce, purify, liquefy, separate ⇨ nutrients, poisons ⇨
b) **Circulation**: absorbed ⇨ **blood** via capillaries (microscopic, porous tubes): *SI, LI* ⇨ arteries, veins (larger, non-porous) ⇨ **heart** ⇨ a/v/c ⇨ all tissues (including blood **cleansing** organs), cells
- Blood carries nutrients, hormones, poisons, etc.
- Total vessels, length > 100,000 miles. Complete circuit of blood, head ⇔ toe: once every 90 sec.
c) Not digested, absorbed ⇨ waste ⇨ **elimination**

4. There are only two **foods, nutrients** (elemental compounds in food): building, cleansing

I. **Building**
*   Build, fuel, thicken, harden, heat, acidify
*   Dry, moisten (grease, mucus)
*   Poison (carbon dioxide, uric acid, ammonia, etc.)

A. Nutrients

1. **Protein** (amino acids): body's primary substance
*   Blood clotting, antibodies, uric acid, cancer
*   Water-soluble, replaced every 6 months

2. **Saturated fat** (fatty acids): all animal, coconut, palm kernel oil, etc. transformed by liver ⇨

3. **Cholesterol** (fatty): all animal
*   Brain, nerves, adrenal glands, hormones, bile.
*   No dietary requirement.

Excess saturated fat, cholesterol ⇨
a) Low density lipoproteins (LDL), "bad cholesterol" transport cholesterol from liver, intestines ⇨ tissues, cells. Excess ⇨ triglycerides, plaque ⇨ thicken, harden the arteries
b) Tumors, stones, obesity, cancer

4. **Unsaturated fat** (essential fatty acids, EFA): fatty fish, seeds, nuts, avocados, olives, etc.
*   Brain, heart, bones, anti-inflammatory
*   High density lipoprotein (HDL), "good" transport cholesterol (arteries) ⇨ liver (dissolve, eliminate); reduce plaque, increase nitric oxide/ gas: relaxes, widens blood vessels, improves blood flow.

B. Food
*   **Animal**: red meat, chicken, turkey (red > white): (high #1, 2, 3) > whole, full-fat dairy > fish (1, 4, low 2, 3), eggs (1, 3, 4, low 2) > low, no fat dairy
*   **Plant**: carbohydrates/ nuts, seeds, beans (1, 4) > grain (sugar, low 1)

II. **Cleansing**
- Watery, airy (gaseous) ⇨ sinks, moves food down
- Cool, moisten, alkalize, purify, laxative, diuretic
- Digest protein, fat; vital to all structure function

A. Nutrients
- **Water**, **minerals**, **vitamins**, protein (enzymes)
- Carbohydrates (sugar, starch, fiber)

B. Food (plant)
- Fruit, vegetables
- Cane sugar, honey, maple syrup, etc.

Every diet: **balance of opposites** (building, cleansing, raw, cooked, etc.) with one opposite always in excess. There are no neutral foods, meals, diets.

HOT, BUILDING, animal, 1- 4 > 5 > 6 > 7, 8
1. **Atkins**: beef, pork, lamb, chicken, fish, eggs
2. **Ketogenic**: red meat, chicken, cheese, berries
3. **Paelo**: red meat, eggs, nuts, seeds, no dairy
4. **South Beach**: bacon, turkey, chicken, eggs
+ Vegetables (leafy greens, roots, ground) +/- fruit
+ Low or no high starch carbs (bread, rice, potatoes)
5. **Pescatarian**: fish, eggs, dairy, vegetables, fruit
6. **Mediterranean**: fish, vegan, olive oil, wine
7. **Macrobiotic**: fish, vegan, miso, seaweed, etc.
8. **Ovo-lacto vegetarian**: eggs, dairy, vegan

COLDER, less BUILDING, animal, more plant/ vegan
9. **Lacto-vegetarian**: dairy, vegan
10. **Vegan**: fruit, vegetables, grains, nuts, beans, seeds, honey, maple syrup, sugar, etc.
11. **Sproutarian**: vegan, raw, sprouts, juices, etc.
12. **Fruitarian**: fruit, juice, water

All food is processed. The best diet can become the worst, disease causing if poorly:
- **Digested** via overeating, meals too close, etc.
- **Eliminated** via overeating, late meals, inactivity

Diets #**1**- **5** high saturated fat, cholesterol: thick, hard, sticky nutrients require greater time, energy, acid, enzymes, bile to process, transport, EASIER when young, lean, unclogged or active; HARDER, disease causing when older (lesser energy, activity), obese, clogged (intestines, arteries) or hot climate (generally less building, animal, more cooling, fruit, vegetables). More vegetarians live in the south than the north.

Diets #**6**- **8**: EASIER. #**9**- **10**: EASIEST, quickest (cooked > raw); disease causing if weak, cold. #**11**- **12**: extreme cleansing, cooling, disease causing if weak, dry.

Correct diet: centered on body's nutrient make-up =
- **1/3 building**: 16% protein, 16% fat (watery)
- **2/3 cleansing**: 64% water, 4% minerals, <1% vitamins ⇨ body (70% water, as Earth)

Greater (>) or lesser (<) nutrients, amounts ⇨ extreme (condition, climate) ⇨ disease. Ayurveda:

Three dietary/ nutrient, energetic disease extremes:
1. Excess building, protein, sat. fat, cholesterol, fire
2. Deficient building, fire, excess air (wind)
3. Excess cleansing, water, sugar, cold drinks, dairy

Treatment plan: diet, herbs (days, months)

Herbs (plant medicine, no protein, fat) are generally necessary as food alone is not powerful enough to prevent or cure all disease. There are only **five** herbs despite variety and number. Each is defined energetically via overall taste (5).
1. Bitter: cold, drying
2. Astringent: cold, drying
3. Sweet: cold, moistening
4. Sour: hot, moistening
5. Pungent (spicy): hot, drying

Herbs supplement, do not replace diet. Most are powerless without corrective diet.

Example: herbs and nutritional supplements that help build bones: ineffective without sufficient protein, fat (chicken, turkey, eggs, dairy, nuts, seeds, beans) ⇨ build, hold the bones, minerals together. Herbs have their limits. Some diseases, conditions will require stronger medicine, M.D., drugs, surgery, etc. None change poor diet, which continues to repeat, sicken in one form, location, or another.

Three dietary, nutritional, energetic diseases:

I. **Excess building** protein, sat. fat, cholesterol via:
- Red meat, pork, turkey, chicken, whole dairy, pizza, butter, oil, chips, etc. ⇨
- Build, thicken, harden, heat, poison, weaken ⇨

A. Clots, plaque, atherosclerosis, arteriosclerosis ⇨
- High blood pressure (hypertension), angina, red face, insomnia, stroke, paralysis, death
- Poor circulation ⇨ head (poor vision, hearing, memory), arms, legs (pain, inflammation, numbness, arthritis); penis (impotence)

B. Acidity, heartburn, GERD, ulcers, stones, UTI
C. Cirrhosis, jaundice, profuse perspiration
D. Acne, psoriasis, gout, foul body odor, migraines
E. Dysmenorrhea, endometriosis, prostatitis, anger
F. Tumors (benign, cancer), rigidity (organs, vessels)

Treatment: Naturopathy (natural medicine):
- Vegetarian #9- 12, bitter, astringent herbs
- Organic beets (anti-tumor), leafy greens (raw or juice): nitrates/ nitric oxide relaxes, widens blood vessels, improves blood, oxygen flow, lowers BP
- +/- M.D.

CASE HISTORIES: majority via health food store (1984- 2001), 70+ customers daily, 6 days/ week. I counseled many (repeat, daily, weekly, years), always asked "What did you eat for breakfast, lunch, dinner, last two days?" More info: About the Author.

#1. 2008 Man (38, obese): chronic **psoriasis** since childhood: dry, scaly, flaky, itchy red skin, prescription drugs. Long-term diet: meat, chicken, cheese, chips, alcohol, smoking. I advised less animal, chips, etc., more fruit, vegetables, organic carrots (snack). Seven months later, he had lost 60 lbs., was cured, had brand new healthy, glowing skin. He also looked 15 yrs. younger.

#2. Two women (60+), past diet (high animal) cured **breast tumors**, **cancer** via vegetarian diet, organic vegetables, beets, bitter herbs: Essiac tea/ Marie Caisse, R.N. via native Indian medicine man (Canada). Both had refused chemotherapy and surgery. Years later, one started eating chicken ⇨ tumor came back ⇨ stopped eating chicken ⇨ 2 months ⇨ tumor disappeared.

#3. I (51): excruciating heel pain, limping, dragging my feet for seven months ⇨ M.D., podiatrist: diagnosed **Plantar Fasciitis**: inflamed, loose ligaments (ankles, feet). His solution, cure: surgery (tighten ligaments), orthotics, drugs, hot, cold compresses. I declined, as his "cure" seemed more like pain management. His diagnosis however, was of great value, helped me figure out the cause: clogged arteries (animal) ⇨ decreased blood ⇨ legs, feet, ligaments ⇨ weak, painful. I cured (4 months) via vegetarian diet, bitter herbs, spices.

 # 4, 5. I (53): obese, overweight (20#), **high blood pressure** (150/110) and **arthritis**, pain, numbness in arms or legs when crossed or raised via narrow arteries, past animal (40's). I changed my diet: vegetarian, more raw vegetables, fruit, juices, spices, etc. Three months later: 20 lb. loss, no pain and BP reduced to 110/70.

II. **Deficient building** protein, fat, animal, plant
- Worsened with salads, juices, cold drinks ⇨
- Thin, dry, cool, air (wind), weaken, loosen ⇨

A. Abdominal bloating, gas, reflux (GIRD)
B. Thin blood, anemia, pallor, fatigue, bruises easily
C. Amenorrhea, PMS, dysmenorrhea, miscarriage

    D. Infertility, impotence, emaciation, palpitations
    E. Thin, dry, shaky, inflamed nerves, muscles, etc.
    F. Arthritis, neuralgia, Plantar Fasciitis, autoimmune
    G. Attention Deficit Disorder, fear, anxiety, cold, flu

Treatment: Naturopathy (East, West)
- Red meat, chicken, eggs, diary, nuts, etc.
- Vegetables (cooked > raw), spices, salt
- +/- M.D.

CASE HISTORIES

#6. 1997 Woman (36, FL): macrobiotic, mostly vegan, low protein, fat, high salads, juices, some cheese ⇨ anemia, deficiency, lack of holding ⇨ **4 miscarriages**. She was seriously deficient, which is why I recommended red meat, chicken or turkey, cooked vegetables, etc. 2x/day + Siberian ginseng, Evening Primrose Oil (blood, sex organs) and waiting 4 mos. (new, greater protein, fat, blood) before trying. She now has two healthy boys.

#7. 2000. Mother: daughter (11), pale, thin, doing poorly in school, diagnosed (M.D.): **Attention Deficit Disorder** ⇨ Adderall, Dexedrine (amphetamines*). School (no psychiatrist, M.D.) wanted to add Ritalin*. Her mother was worried. Her daughter looked anemic. I questioned her daughter about her diet. Did she like red meat, chicken, vegetables (which ones?), etc. = solution. Yes. I recommended the diet (breakfast, dinner); school (lunch her choice) and more personal attention. Six months later, I received a letter with a report card (all A's, 1 B, math) thanking me.

#8. Woman (65, vegetarian, S. FL): frequent **anxiety** (fear, worry, nervousness, irritability, sweating) screaming and yelling at me or her husband from one anxiety attack to another during consultation; incontinence, etc. My initial impression: excess heat, however there was no excess fuel. She was suffering deficiency (blood, protein, fat) ⇨ weakness, lack of confidence, control but instead anxiety, fear, worry, for a person who was always strong, successful, positive.

I recommended animal (meat, chicken, eggs), cooked vegetables, spices, etc. Problem: vegetarian. I told her it was a matter of life and death. She compromised, veal, eggs. Three days later, she called. "Is this the genius?" She was very happy, no anxiety, having great bowel movements and teaching her employees deep abdominal breathing, which I had taught her during consultation to calm her down.

#9. Woman (26, athlete), **neuralgia**: severe foot pain (walking, standing), numerous doctors, blood specialists, orthopedic surgeons, acupuncturists, chiropractors, blood work, x-rays, MRI, etc. to no avail. I (two min.) diagnosed anemia via long-term low protein, fat diet, starting teens ⇨ weakness, neuralgia I recommended red meat, cooked vegetables, etc. every day. A year later, 80%, she was better, could stand, walk, exercise without pain or fear. She cured fully when she decided to eat red meat 2x/ day.

   III. **Excess water, sugar** via water, fruit, juice, smoothies, sugar (natural, synthetic), soda, beer, cold drinks, raw vegetables ⇨

   A. Cool, moisten, dilute, weaken acid, enzymes ⇨

   1. Stomach, small intestine ⇨ indigestion, bloating, gas, reflux, malabsorption

   2. Large intestine ⇨ indigestion, bloating, gas, loose stools

   B. Water, sugar ⇨ SI, LI, capillaries ⇨ blood ⇨

   1. Kidneys, urinary bladder ⇨ excessive urine, urination, urinary tract, yeast infection

   2. Cellulite, edema, coldness

   3. Excess sugar weakens salivary glands ⇨ decreases saliva (moistens mouth) ⇨ dry mouth

Treatment: Naturopathy
- Grains, beans, vegetables (cooked > raw)
- Spices (hot), bitter, astringent herbs
- +/- M.D.

#10. Woman (35): **Irritable Bowel Syndrome**: bloating, gas, nausea, loose stools, swollen arms (3x normal) via dairy, salads, juices, etc. I recommended grains, beans, cooked vegetables, spices +/- chicken. Nine months later, all symptoms gone but still worried ⇨ nutritionist ($300) ⇨ stool sample (excess bacteria) ⇨ **golden seal** (bitter, cold, antibacterial), nine caps/ day. She came to my store 3 weeks later to buy more. I asked why, how long, results? All gastrointestinal symptoms returned. I explained. **Bitter herbs** generally kill healthy digestive bacteria. 9 caps/ day: extreme, appropriate: edema, infections (which she did not have), not someone cold, weak digestion, still recovering, which is why she reacted so poorly. I refused the sale, had her continue the original diet, spices, etc. She recovered.

#11. Woman (35, trim), **cellulite** via dairy, salads, juices, cold drinks. I advised cooked vegetables, beans, spices, bitter herbs, no dairy, which decreased cellulite.

4. Lungs, nose, sinuses ⇨ water, mucus, phlegm ⇨
- Coughing, sinusitis, sleep apnea, colds, flu
- Viruses thrive in stagnant water, mucus
- Winter, cold air slows, thickens fluids ⇨ mucus

Common cold, flu (viruses). U.S.A. (330 million):
- Every year: 40% vaccinated
- 10% (33 million) mostly unvaccinated catch the flu: mild, low death rate until COVID
- The rest (includes 40%) generally do not

2020: COVID, no vaccine, except normal flu (40%)
- 30 million sick (9%), 400,000 deaths (1.3%)
- #3 (death): majority (obese, heart disease) *
- 60% unvaccinated: did not get or report sick

2021: COVID vaccine: same number

2022: COVID (60% vaccinated)
- 30 million (9%) sick, 300,000 deaths *

World (8 billion): 250 million COVID cases/ year: 3%

U.S.A. despite "best" doctors, technology, shutdown, isolation: #1: COVID infections, deaths. Real epidemic: poor diet, obesity (35% adults, 20% children), heart disease, lack of prevention, education more so than a lack of health care, waiting to get sick and then acting.

Flu vaccine (per strain): generally safe, effective, provides short-term (4-6 months) answer, protection, but does not exercise, strengthen long-term immunity, change diet, lifestyle, etc. Treatment: CH. 20 (Cold, Flu)

Not everyone who is exposed catches the flu, gets sick. The majority who are flu resistant, do not catch or quickly cure, are young, healthy, lean or active. Better health (#12) is the answer.

#12. I (73) lacto-vegetarian (+/- vegan) since age 51, spices (age 37). Last 46 years: no flu shots (personal choice), **colds, flus** or fever (indicates viral infection) but instead occasional coughs, sore throats that were cured quickly (onset, day 1- 2) via vegetable soup, spices, herbs: cardamom, ginger, licorice (sore throat).

Everyone, everything (condition, diet, climate, etc.) changes. Today's diet may improve health but tomorrow worsen, and vice versa. The proof is always the outcome. Eat what works for you. Be flexible, patient, and wise. Do not harm yourself for dietary goals.

Extreme dietary changes ⇨ overwhelm, sicken.

Case history #15 (1981): I was the "camp "doctor" at a macrobiotic summer camp (Amherst, MA).

Many attendees were not macrobiotic nor strict vegetarian. The menu was too strict: vegan, limited desserts (fruit). Two days later, a woman came to me crying and wanting to leave. I recommended she go into town, eat whatever she wanted and then decide. She went, had pizza, ice cream, coffee and came back happy, stayed. I reported this to my superiors, who added fish, more desserts to the menu.

Herbs, generally harmless can be misused, harm.

Case history #13.

1. 1992 (42, lean, active): my own liver cleansing formula: too much bupleurum (bitter) ⇨ dried, contracted lungs ⇨ night ⇨ wake up, gasping.

2. 2013 (61, lacto-vegetarian) added bitter herbs, coffee (bitter). A few months later after a few beers (bitter) ⇨ red face, dizziness, nausea, rapid heartbeat, angina, fever. I stopped the bitters, coffee and cured. Three days later, all my hair ⇨ top ⇨ sides ⇨ back ⇨ brittle, broke off. I consulted a nurse: diagnosed anemia ⇨ hair loss. I started eating red meat, chicken: high iron. Heart symptoms returned. I eliminated animal, bitters, increased dairy. My hair grew back.

Herbs have limits, which is why allopathic medicine (drugs, surgery etc.) may be necessary, as it is quicker, more powerful, and many times life-saving.

1. Man tried curing **poison ivy rash** with herbs. I first saw him on day 5: arm swollen, skin, shiny, bright red. I told him that his condition was serious, life-threatening: infection could pass into blood. He needed to see an M.D. which he did. The doctor verified the severity, prescribed drugs, which cured, saved his life.

2. I (26), severe **tonsillitis, strep throat** tried to cure via macrobiotic diet, herbs, acupuncture to no avail. I got worse, almost died. An M.D., penicillin saved my life (About the Author).

Allopathy while powerful is an emergency medicine that kills disease to improve health. It also harms. Johns Hopkins study (2019): **iatrogenic**, physician induced disease: 3rd leading cause of death (300,000). U.S.A. despite "best" doctors, medical care ranks:

- 26th out of 35 (world's democracies) in longevity
- 5th highest cancer, heart disease, diabetes, infant mortality rates
- Only 1 of 3 out of 35 that allow pharmaceutical advertising on television

Case history #14. Several elderly customers: diuretics (water pills) for high blood pressure ⇨ years ⇨ bones (hands, feet) ⇨ thin, melted, fused. Diuretics increase calcium secretion ⇨ decreases bone mineral density ⇨ extreme ⇨ fractures. My brother's lower leg fractured one day while standing.

Exercise increases respiration, expansion, contraction, movement, blood, oxygen, circulation, digestion, elimination, etc.

Sexual essence (sperm, ovum, hormones): body's vital but limited (you get one fuel tank) substance (high protein, fat), fuel for all structure, function ⇨

1. **Fountain of youth**, health, power, when full

2. **Aging**, dryness, weakness, physical, mental decline, starts: men (late teens), women (early 20's). Moderation (sex) ⇨ health, longevity.

Body, physical health, power, pleasure is nice but does not last but instead naturally declines with time. Most importantly, it does not guarantee lasting happiness, which is the greatest health, pleasure, power.

Nor do family, friends, job, money, power, etc. guarantee lasting happiness, as all decline, become boring or pass away with time, always end in pain, loss, disappointment, depression, anger, etc.

Life is body, mind and spirit (Spirit). The spirit has its own structures, functions, **seven chakras** (spiritual energy centers in the brain, spine), maintenance plan, **spiritual practices** (meditation, prayer, kindness, generosity, vegetarian diet, fasting, celibacy, morality, study, love of God, etc.) ⇨ supernatural **powers** (control of elements, matter, energy), **pleasures**, never-ending joy, peace, etc. is the future promise, advertised message of God via many religions, more so in the East than West.

Most people who believe in God believe in a heaven (kingdom of God), better, joyous after-life (greater than this life). "The kingdom of God is within you." Luke 17:21.

Just as energy exists within, creates matter, so does spirit (consciousness) exist within, create energy.

The more the mind concentrates, attaches itself to the **spirit** (Spirit/ God), the greater health, happiness. The lesser attachment, greater attachment to anything else, the greater disease, pain, suffering.

Life is body, mind and spirit (soul). It is foolish not to take advantage, use all the parts and tools available. The rules, rewards and punishments are the same for everyone.

"To know is to do, and to do is to know."

1. NUTRITION, DIET

BODY: 30 trillion cells ⇨ **tissues**: 3 trillion nerves, 7 glands, 10 organs, muscles; **vessels**: arteries, veins, capillaries; **fluids**: hormones, blood, antibodies, etc. are created, increased, decreased, heated, cooled, dried, aired, moistened, poisoned, cleansed or destroyed daily via diet: food (animal, plant), nutrients. There are only two: building, cleansing.

Correct diet, balance, kinds, amounts ⇨ health (normal structure function) is centered on the body's constitution, nutrient make-up, balance:
- **1/3 building** (32% protein, fat): animal, plant
- **2/3 cleansing** (64% water, 4% minerals, <1% vitamins): fruit, vegetables
- Greater (**>**) or lesser (**<**) foods, nutrients, amounts ⇨ **extreme** (varies) ⇨ disease

All **food** ⇨ **processed** (transformed, transported) ⇨

1. Stomach ⇨ small intestine (24' tube) ⇨ large intestine (5', sac, tube) ⇨ acid, enzymes, bile, bacteria/ flora ⇨ **digest**, heat, reduce, liquefy, purify, separate ⇨ nutrients, fiber, poisons ⇨

2. Absorbed ⇨ **blood** (92% water) via capillaries (microscopic porous tubes) in SI, LI ⇨ **circulated** ⇨ arteries, veins (larger, non-porous) ⇨ heart ⇨ arteries, capillaries (10 billion) ⇨ all tissues, cells.
- Total vessels, length > 100,000 miles.
- Complete circuit: blood, head ⇔ toe once every 90 seconds.

3. Not digested, absorbed ⇨ waste ⇨ **elimination**

BODY: 64% water, 65% oxygen. Its major structures, tissues: normally **spongey**, thick, thin, watery, solid, hollow, interconnected ⇨ continual movement, easy exchange, absorption, elimination of blood, nutrients, hormones, poisons, etc.in, out every cell.

Quality and quantity of food, nutrients affect positively and negatively, slow, weaken transformation and transportation, digestion, circulation, cleansing, etc.

I. **Building**

A. Nutrients (elemental compounds in food)
- Build, moisten (grease, mucus), thicken, harden
- Fuel, heat, acidify, poison (uric acid, ammonia, carbon dioxide, etc.)

1. **Protein** (amino acids): body's primary substance
- Organs, glands, nerves, bones, enzymes
- Hormones, antibodies, clots, uric acid (gout)
- 20 amino acids. Nine essential (supplied via diet) Animal: complete, all 9, well balanced. Plants: no. Combining grains with beans, nuts or seeds = 9.
- Water-soluble, replaced every 6 months

2. **Saturated fat** (fatty acids): all animal, coconut, palm kernel oil; beans, nuts (low)
- Need declines after age two (varies)
- Transformed by liver ⇨
3. **Cholesterol** (fatty): brain, nerves, adrenal glands, hormones, bile. No dietary requirement.

Excess saturated fat, cholesterol (all animal) ⇨
- Low density lipoproteins (**LDL**), "bad cholesterol" ⇨ plaque ⇨ arteries ⇨ heart.
- Tumors, stones, obesity
- +/- **trans fats** (hydrogenated oils): butter, full-fat dairy, fried foods, processed meats, sugar ⇨ triglycerides ⇨ arteriosclerosis, pancreatitis

4. **Unsaturated fat** (essential fatty acids, EFA): fatty fish (Omega 3): brain, heart, bones, skin; seed, nuts, avocados, olives (Omega 6): anti-inflammatory + brain, heart, etc.
- High density lipoproteins (**HDL**), "good" reduce plaque, relax, widen vessels, improve blood flow.

All fat: high energy (7 calories/ gram). Sugar (4)

Food (animal, plant)

1. **Red meat** highest protein, sat. fat, cholesterol (avoid pork: impure, omnivore, sweet = pus) >>
2. **Chicken, turkey** (red > white meat) >>
3. **Fish** low saturated fat, cholesterol, high EFA #3 (wild, farmed: +/- mercury, fecal contamination)

4. **Eggs** high protein, cholesterol, EFA #3, 6, low sat fat), unfertilized not considered flesh >>>

5. **Dairy**: best quality: raw, unpasteurized, hormone, antibiotic free, alive, easily absorbable nutrients, digestive enzymes. U.S., 9 million users, legal (17 states): low sickness, death (rare).
- Pasteurization kills most vitamins, enzymes, bacteria, which is why most milk is "fortified."

a) **Hard cheese**: protein, saturated fat, cholesterol, salt, calcium, mucus. Swiss cheese (least) >>>
b) **Butter, heavy cream** (high sat. fat, cholesterol, low calcium) >>> **cottage cheese** >>
c) **Milk** (whole: high sat. fat, cholesterol >> low or no fat*), best digested alone, lightly boiled + ginger, cardamom, +/- whole grains, bananas, papayas.
d) **Yogurt** (sour, hot, beneficial bacteria): high calcium, magnesium, potassium, digests well with vegetables, cucumber, cardamom, coriander, cumin, cilantro; poorly: milk, nuts, sour fruit.
e) **Ice cream** (dietary nightmare): cold, sugar, fat

Green plants (#6- 9, fruit, vegetables, honey, etc.):
a) Protein, fat, minerals, vitamins, enzymes, oxygen
b) Carbohydrates:
- Sugar (grain, fruit, vegetables, honey, etc.): body's main energy source (4cal./gm.) ⇨ glucose.
- Fiber/ starch (#6- 9, fruit, vegetables): reduces cholesterol absorption; slows sugar absorption
c) High solar radiation, electrical currents support nerves. Animal (2nd hand, lesser).

6. **Beans** (mung, azuki, chickpea, lentil, tofu, etc.): protein, EFA (#6), starch, drying, acidic

7. **Nuts** (almonds, walnuts, pine nuts, etc.): protein, EFA (#6), minerals, best raw, ground*

8. **Seeds** (sesame, flax, etc.): protein, EFA (#6), minerals; complete nutrition of grown plant *

9. **Grains**: vit. B, E, minerals, sugar, protein, fiber
- Whole: more nutritious, vital >> cracked >> flour
- Popped, flour, yeast: drying
- Diuretic: barley, quinoa, millet, corn, buckwheat
- Acidic: with animal, fruit, sugar or not thoroughly chewed, mixed with saliva (alkaline)

II. **Cleansing**
- Watery, airy (gaseous) ⇨ sinks, moves food down
- Cool, moisten, alkalize, purify, dissolve
- Digest protein, fat, cholesterol, paste; laxative
- Support all biochemical activities

A. Nutrients
- **Water, minerals, vitamins** (water, fat-soluble)
- Protein (enzymes), carbs (sugar, starch/ fiber)

B. Food (plant)

1. **Fruit**: high water, enzymes, vitamins, sugar
- Air (wind): especially dried; cranberries (diuretic)
- Tropical (hot, damp, mucus), juices (mucus)
- Digests well: beginning of meal (Ayurveda); poorly (gas, acidity): end, +/- beans, grains, sugar

2. **Vegetables**: high minerals, vitamins, enzymes, fiber, water, less sugar. Three kinds.

a) Above ground: leaf
- Collard greens, kale, spinach, lettuce, carrot tops, watercress: high chlorophyl, nitrates
- Cleanses, cools, oxygenates
- Upper body: lungs, heart + liver (LV), intestines

b) Ground level: round, stalks
- Hard squashes, onions: sweet, heavy, grounding
- Broccoli, cauliflower, celery, cabbage: gaseous
- Cleanses middle abdomen: ST, SP, P, LV, GB

c) Below ground: roots
- Beets, carrots, burdock, parsnips, turnips, etc.
- Sweet, cool, fibrous, cleanse
- Lower abdomen: SI, LI, kidneys, UB, sex organs

Preparation:
1. **Raw**: high Vit. B, C, nitrates, cooling, cleansing, gaseous; best consumed at end of meal.
2. **Cooked**: hotter, less water-soluble nutrients (Vit. B, C), more starch, but better digestion, nutrient absorption via breakdown of cellular walls
3. **Fermented** vegetables, grains, beans: salty, sour, heating, increase digestion, saliva, appetite
- Too much ⇨ thirst, acidity, swollen liver, rashes

Seaweed nori, arame, kelp, wakame, kombu, hijiki
- High minerals: calcium (10x dairy), iodine (I), salt
- Sedates, softens, dissolves (phlegm, fibroids)
- Too much increases swelling, blood pressure

Spirulina (blue green algae/ bacteria) grows in fresh water via photosynthesis. Best quality: organic. Harvested (wild): toxic, heavy metals ⇨ liver damage
- High vitamins, minerals, chlorophyl, antioxidant
- Detoxifies, removes heavy metals; cooling
- Lowers BP, cholesterol; increases antibodies

Sugar (saccharide): energy source (calories) via diet (fruit, vegetables, grain, sugar (natural, synthetic etc.) helps build RNA, DNA, etc.

Excessive sugar: concentrated, natural, synthetic ⇨
1. Obesity, diabetes, scarring of the liver
2. Binds to protein and lipids (fat) ⇨
- Reduces skin plasticity, flexibility, depletes collagen ⇨ aging, inflammation

3. Sugar + protein ⇨ oxygen radicals ⇨ aging
4. Excessive sugar ⇨ **triglycerides** (page 24)

Organically grown produce, food, herbs:
- Natural fertilizers (grass, manure, etc.)
- No artificial chemicals, fertilizers, preservatives, dyes, additives, insecticides, herbicides, etc.
- Best quality food, nutrition, taste, healing

Large corporate farms: high artificial chemicals, fertilizers, etc. year in year out depletes, poisons the soil. Organic farming: alternates, rests fields (1 year) ⇨ rejuvenate naturally ⇨ healthy. Smaller farms generally use lesser sprays. Washing, boiling eliminates external water-soluble poisons but not internal. Discard cooking water (poisons) unless organic.

Water cools, moistens and facilitates all function. Best quality: spring or running (not bottled), room temperature. Most residential water is contaminated (chemicals, bacteria). Good filters remove 98%+. Avoid distilled (leaches minerals), exception: kidney stones.

Salt (rock, sea, etc.): essential to life. Body (blood), oceans: same salt content. Body, earth: 70% water.
- Anabolic, laxative, increases digestion, salivation
- Moistens, softens, dissolves phlegm, tumors
- Excess ⇨ dry skin, wrinkles, edema, rashes, arteriosclerosis, high blood pressure, ulcer

Every meal, diet: balance of opposites (building, cleansing, hot, cold, raw, cooked, etc.) with one opposite always in excess. There are no neutral meals, diets.

HOT, BUILDING, animal, 1- 4 > 5 > 6 > 7, 8
1. **Atkins**: beef, pork, lamb, chicken, fish, eggs
2. **Ketogenic**: red meat, chicken, cheese, berries
3. **Paelo**: red meat, eggs, nuts, seeds, no dairy
4. **South Beach**: bacon, turkey, chicken, eggs
+ Vegetables (leafy greens, roots, ground) +/- fruit
+ Low or no high starch carbs (bread, rice, potatoes)
5. **Pescatarian**: fish, eggs, dairy, vegetables, fruit

6. **Mediterranean**: fish, vegan, olive oil, wine
7. **Macrobiotic**: vegan, fermented foods + fish
8. **Ovo-lacto vegetarian**: eggs, dairy, vegan

COLDER, less BUILDING, animal, more plant/ vegan
9. **Lacto-vegetarian**: dairy, vegan
10. **Vegan**: fruit, vegetables (land, sea), grains, nuts beans, seeds, honey, maple syrup, sugar, etc.
11. **Sproutarian**: vegan, raw, sprouts, juices
12. **Fruitarian**: fruit, juice, water

All food, fluids ⇨ processed ⇨ digested, absorbed, circulated, cleansed, etc. Some foods, nutrients (building) are thicker, harder to process, more disease causing. Others (cleansing) are easier, thinner, watery.

Diets #**1- 5** high saturated fat, cholesterol require greater time, energy and fuel to digest, cleanse, circulate, easier when young or active; harder, disease causing when older, obese, clogged (intestines, arteries), inactive or living in hot climate. #**6- 8**: easier.

Diets #**9- 10**: easiest, quickest (cooked > raw); disease causing when weak, cold. #**11- 12**: extreme cleansing, cooling, disease causing when weak, cold, dry.

General rules: digestion (CH. 7), nutrient absorption:

1. The **more** you eat per or between meals (<4 hrs. apart), the **lesser** digestion, absorption; greater bloating, waste, weight. Smaller meals: greater digestion, absorption, weight control.
   - No written rule: 3 meals/ day. 2 meals + snacks may suffice when older, less active.
   - "To lengthen thy life, lessen thy meals."

2. TCM, Ayurveda: digestive organs strongest, highly charged: **9 A.M. – 3 P.M**: sun + greater activity, upright posture ⇨ moves food down, increases mixing, acid, enzymes, etc.
   - Night: less active, more sitting, laying down ⇨ food stagnation, bloating, gas, malabsorption

- Eat like a king (biggest meal: protein, fat, vegetables, etc.) for breakfast, queen (lesser) for lunch, prince, pauper (least) for dinner.

3. Spices (hot > mild) stimulate stomach, pancreas, small intestine, liver, acid, enzymes, bile ⇨ increase digestion, nutrient absorption.

4. Bitter herbs stimulate liver, release of bile digest fat, increases peristalsis (muscular contractions of SI, LI ⇨ moves food, stools down).

5. Excess fluids with meals dilute, weaken digestion.

6. Regular eating times train, strengthen digestive organs. Irregular times weaken.

Correct diet is centered on the body's constitution, nutrient make-up, balance:
- **1/3 building** (32% protein, fat): animal, plant
- **2/3 cleansing** (64% water, 4% minerals, <1% vitamins): fruit, vegetables
- Greater (**>**) or lesser (**<**) amounts, kinds ⇨ **extreme** (days, years) ⇨ disease

Ayurveda: **three** dietary, nutritional, energetic disease extremes:
  I.   Excess building (animal > plant), fire
  II. Deficient building (animal, plant), excess air
  III. Excess water, sugar (natural, synthetic), cold, fruit, juices, sodas, smoothies, cold drinks, air

Treatment plan: do more of the opposite until healthy
  1. Excess building: less building, more cleansing
  2. Deficient building: more building
  3. Excess water, cold: less water, more fire, drying

Herbs (plant medicine, no protein, fat) are generally necessary as food alone is not powerful enough to prevent or cure most disease. Diet, herbs generally take time (days, months) to cure, if curable via diet, herbs.

There are only five herbs (CH. 3), each defined according to overall taste (5) and energy. Some herbs may conflict with prescription drugs. Consult an M.D.

1. Bitter: cold, dry, airy, cleansing, depletes energy

2. Astringent: cold, dry, airy, cleansing

3. Sweet: cold, moist, holds, increases energy

4. Sour: hot, moist, holds, increases energy

5. Pungent (spices): hot, dry, airy, cleansing

Recommended, middle diet meal plan:
- Central theme: 1/3 building, 2/3 cleansing
- Three treatment plans, variations + herbs
- 1- 3 meals per day, except animal food (2)
- Treatment time: days, months

I. **Excess building**

A. Red meat, turkey, chicken, fish, eggs, hard cheese, butter, protein, sat. fat, cholesterol ⇨
- Thicken, harden, heat, poison, weaken ⇨

1. Blood clots, high cholesterol, LDL ⇨ plaque ⇨ thickens, narrows, clogs arteries, heart ⇨

- Reduced circulation, blood, nutrients ⇨ arms, legs ⇨ dryness, inflammation, pain, stiffness, arthritis

- High blood pressure, palpitations, tachycardia
- Angina, insomnia, heart attack, paralysis
- Heart disease #1 cause death (20%): age 65+

2. Gout, stones (kidney, gall), dysuria, UTI
3. PMS, dysmenorrhea, endometriosis, impotence

4. Swollen liver, spleen, distended upper abdomen
5. Jaundice, anemia, pancreatitis, tumors
6. Acne, rashes, psoriasis, warts; cancer

Treatment: **colder middle diet #1**
- Less building, more sweet, watery, cold, drying
- **25% Protein, fat**: milk (low or no fat), soft cheese (no salt), beans
- **25% Grain**: wheat berry, barley, quinoa, basmati rice, oats, granola
- **40% Vegetables**: 3-5/ meal: raw (lettuce, spinach, celery, cabbage, parsley, beets, carrots, sprouts) > cooked (cauliflower, green beans, broccoli, mushrooms, asparagus); Avoid chard, spinach, nightshades, tomatoes (high) peppers
- **10% Fruit**: all, except dried (vata, air) or lemons, limes, bananas, grapefruit (worsen ulcers, UTI) in moderation, seasonal, do not mix
- **Beverages**: water (spring), 3- 4 glasses per day, tea: chamomile, green, raspberry leaf, dandelion
- **Spices** (mild): coriander, fennel, cumin, turmeric
- **Sweeteners**: all (except sugar) unless diabetic
- **Tastes**, **herbs**: sweet, bitter, astringent
- +/- M.D.

Beets (raw or juice), leafy greens: high nitrates ⇨ body ⇨ nitric oxide (vasodilator) ⇨ relaxes, widens blood vessels, lowers blood pressure, improves blood flow, oxygen to muscles, all structure.

Golden seal root: bitter, astringent
- Antibiotic, anti- inflammatory/ tumor/ cancer
- Increases bile, laxative, diuretic
- Detoxifies, cleanses blood, lymph, liver, drugs
- Reduces infection, yeast, hepatitis, jaundice
- Dysmenorrhea, menorrhagia, leukorrhea, obesity
- Avoid if thin, dry, smoker, pregnant

B. Excess flour: pretzels, chips, cookies, bread ⇨ paste, thicken, narrow, clog SI, LI ⇨
- Bloating, acidity, reflux, nausea, malabsorption

Treatment:
- Eliminate flour, increase vegetables, water (+++), fruit, juice: days, weeks

II. **Deficient building** (animal, plant)
- Cool, dry, thin, air, slow, weaken ⇨

Deficient blood (low protein, fat, iron), anemia ⇨
- Fatigue, pallor, cold hands, feet; autoimmune
- Thin, dry, cracked skin, lips, nails, emaciation
- Easily bruises, bleeds, purpura (skin: blood spots)
- Thin, dry, airy nerves, muscles, tendons, etc. ⇨ inflammation, pain, shaking, numbness
- Amenorrhea, PMS, dysmenorrhea, infertility
- Miscarriage, impotence, premature ejaculation
- Frigidity, low libido, fear, anxiety, colds, flus
- Low blood pressure, palpitations, tinnitus (low)
- Premature aging, dementia
- Children: poor mental development, learning disorders via too little EFA

Treatment: **hotter middle diet**
- Building, moistening, heating, grounding
- **30% Protein, fat**: 70% buttermilk, ghee, chicken, turkey, fish, eggs, 30% raw, ground nuts (almonds, walnuts, pecans, pine nuts, etc.), seeds (sesame) +/- red meat (condition, climate)
- **20% Grain** wheat, oats, rice, cous cous
- **40% Vegetables** cooked (+ sesame, avocado, olive, oil): onions, potatoes (sweet, yams, white), carrots, beets, parsley, avocado, radish, seaweed, turnips, green beans; chilies
- **10% fruit**: avoid dried, melons, cranberries
- **Spices** all (except peppers) 3- 7/ meal
- **Sweeteners** all, except white sugar (diabetes)
- **Herbs** sweet (saw palmetto, marshmallow), sour (amla, hawthorn berry)
- **Beverages** water (+/- lemon, lime), milk, sour fruit juices
- +/- M.D.

Amla (amalaki) fruit: sour, cooling, sweet
- Rejuvenative: blood, bones, heart, eyes, teeth
- Anemia, bleeding, osteoporosis, diabetes
- Premature greying, hair loss; mental disorders

Hawthorn berry: sour, heating
- Increases digestion, weight, strengthens heart
- Dissolves food masses, tumors: digestive tract

Saw palmetto berry: sweet, oily, astringent
- Increases nutrient absorption
- Reduces swelling: prostate, ovary, uterus

III. **Excess water**, **sugar**, dairy, juice, cold drinks
- Watery, cold symptoms, diseases

- Weak digestion bloating, gas, malabsorption
- Lungs ⇨ excess water, mucus ⇨ congestion ⇨ sinusitis, coughing, shortness of breath, asthma
- Kidneys, urinary bladder ⇨ excessive urination
- Edema, cellulite, obesity, diabetes, yeast, UTI

Treatment: **colder middle diet #2**
- **30% Protein, fat** beans: adzuki, soy, lima, lentils, etc.; soymilk, buttermilk +/- nuts, seeds, white meat chicken, turkey (condition, climate)
- **30% Grain** barley, quinoa, dried grains, corn
- **40% Vegetables** cooked broccoli, cabbage, celery, chilies, carrots, green beans, radishes, watercress, asparagus, mushrooms, raw sprouts, lettuce: **fruit** minimal: dried (all), cranberry, apple
- **Sweeteners** raw honey (astringent)
- **Spices** (all) 3- 7/ meal: ginger, black pepper, cardamom, cinnamon turmeric, garlic, etc.
- **Tea** dandelion, chicory, cinnamon, ginger
- **Tastes**, **herbs** pungent, bitter, astringent
- +/- M.D.

Ginger: pungent, sweet; fresh root (cooler)
- Improves digestion, circulation, immunity
- Settles stomach, moves obstructions (ST, SI)
- Eliminates mucus, phlegm, reduces bloating
- Antiviral, antibacterial, antiseptic

Horsetail: bitter, astringent, sweet
- Diuretic, blood cleanser, regulates minerals

- Reduces infection (mouth, gums, throat), enteritis, cystitis, vaginitis, prostatitis, gonorrhea, edema
- Strengthens bones, dissolves stones

Additional factors affecting diet.

1. **Climate**

- Cold climate generally requires more building, heating, animal, cooking, less cold, raw, juices.

- Hot climate generally less animal, more plant, cooling, cleansing.

- Dry climate more moistening. Damp more drying.

2. **Biology**

a) Length of intestines, mouth to anus: 10-12x length of body like <u>frugivorous</u> animals: eat fruit, vegetables, nuts, grains and not:
- <u>Carnivorous</u> (meat): 3-5x: quicker digestion, elimination, prevents putrefaction
- <u>Herbivorous</u> (grass, plants): 20-28x
- <u>Omnivorous</u> (eats all): length varies

b) Teeth (32): same height
- 20 molars (grinding grains, nuts, seeds, beans)
- 8 incisors (cutting: vegetables, fruit, herbs)
- <u>4 canines (tearing: flesh)</u> =
  32 28: 4 = 7 (plant): 1 (animal)

- <u>Frugivore</u>: same height, mostly molars, incisors
- <u>Carnivore</u>: canines most developed, long, sharp, smooth, pointed, molars are pointed
- <u>Omnivore</u>: canines (carnivore), incisors herbivore
- <u>Herbivore</u>: incisors well developed, canines stunted, molars broad-topped

c) Lactase (digestive enzyme via small intestine) digests lactose (dairy sugar)

d) **Blood type** (4): A, B, AB, O. Each has its own dietary likes, dislikes. Blood type: constitutional diagnosis, treatment plan which does not change unlike condition, which does. Vegetarian diet (lower protein, fat) benefits type A, especially those who suffer excess protein, fat diseases but may worsen A's, low protein, fat diseases, live in a cold climate.

3. General longevity, health (world) = vegetarian

Vegetarian diets do not always work. I have counseled vegans (20's, 30's) suffering fatigue, anemia, infertility, miscarriage, impotence, neuralgia, cracked nails, cold, flus, etc. despite nutritionally correct, organic diet, flax seeds, soy protein, spirulina, etc. I recommended animal: meat, chicken, eggs, dairy, etc. Those who ate animal got better (#II).

Case history #16 I (early 20's, healthy, active): severe weight loss, colds, flus, premature ejaculation, impotence, etc. the more vegan, raw I became. I got better via macrobiotic diet. More info: About the Author.

Case history #17 (store). Man (30's): impotent last four months: new girlfriend (vegan). He had stopped eating meat, chicken, etc. became weak, impotent. I advised dairy, eggs and then make a gradual transition or not.

Some people need animal, others not. Everything changes. Sometimes the timing, condition (age, activity, sex, etc.), climate is just not right.

Not eating animal at the expense, sacrifice of one's health, life (higher life-form) is foolish. Story: two Buddhist monks, strict vegans traveling in the woods for four days, had not find any food (fruit, nuts, roots), were starving, cold, shivering, sitting around a fire, when a bird suddenly flew into the fire, followed by another, both dying instantaneously.

The birds were offering themselves (lower life-form) as food for a higher life-form. The monks ate the birds. The moral of the story: man should never sacrifice himself for a lower life-form, as he has a duty to live, spiritually grow into a higher life-form, to help all.

The vegetarian diet is considered spiritual:

1. No killing of animals.

2. Less heating, stimulating to the body, makes it easier to focus on the spirit, unlike animal food (meat, chicken, turkey, fish, eggs, etc.), heavier, more stimulating ⇨ increases body consciousness, sexual desire, etc.

The vegetarian diet, however does not make one a better, more spiritual person. Spiritual, loving thoughts and actions are the guarantor of spiritual development.

Fasting, limited diet: water, fruit, juice ⇨

1. Cleanses excess protein, fat, poisons, waste

2. Accesses prana (CH. 5, 29, 30): body's vital energy, life-force (brain, spine): far greater than food, water, or air, which is why many experience greater energy after 2nd day of fasting

Initial fasts: one day/ week. Longer fasts, 3 days+ generally require supervision.

All fasts: start and end with light diet: soup, cooked vegetables. Avoid heavy foods shortly thereafter (nausea, vomiting). More info: About the Author, p. 308

Recommended: **Miracle of Fasting: Proven Throughout History**, Paul Bragg

Everyone (condition, climate) is different, changes which is why there is no one universal, consistent diet, cure-all.

The same foods, herbs that help heal one person, cure one disease may worsen another. Today's diet may harm but tomorrow heal and vice versa.

Eat what works, makes you happy. Avoid extreme dietary changes (meat, vegetarian), which can build or cleanse too fast ⇨ overwhelm, sicken the body, mind. Positive mental attitude ("I can succeed"), moderation, patience, and flexibility are required as it took time (weeks, years) to get sick and therefore time to cure. Negative attitude undermines any healing modality.

Diet and herbs do not always cure. **Severity may require an M.D.**, drugs, etc. Do not be foolish.

Modern, allopathic medicine (drugs, surgery, etc.) has its value, especially when all else fails. I was foolish, tried curing tonsillitis with diet, herbs and acupuncture. I got worse, almost died. More info: About the Author.

Doing it yourself, shopping, cooking in your own kitchen is your best health insurance, control. Ignore the kitchen and you will most likely not ignore doctors, drugs, hospitalization, suffering, poverty, etc.

2. VITAMINS, MINERALS, ENZYMES

Enzymes, minerals, vitamins, ⇨
- Cool, moisten, thin, alkalize, cleanse, purify
- Digest, assimilate protein, fat, carbohydrates
- Anti-oxidant, support all structure function
- Iron: largest mineral in red blood cells/ hemoglobin: transports oxygen

Nutritional deficiencies, diseases generally indicate larger deficiencies via poor diet and are best corrected via better diet. Nutritional supplements do have short-term benefits, but do not replace much less equal the vitality, nutrition of fruit, vegetables, nuts, seeds, etc. grown in the Earth under the sun, and not in a laboratory.

General use:

1. Capsule (no fillers), powder or liquid: better than tablets with food

2. Short-term, exceptions

3. Best quality: whole foods (yeast, spirulina, wheat germ, etc.): more vital, nutritious than synthetic

4. May conflict with prescription drugs. Ask M.D.

VITAMINS

a) Water-soluble (B complex, C): not stored, taken daily, heat sensitive, destroyed by cooking
b) Fat-soluble (A, D, E, K): stored, live longer, digested via liver bile not destroyed by cooking

Vitamin A (carotenoids)
- Eyes, skin, immune system, bones, teeth
- Antioxidant: protects body from free radicals ⇨ damages cells ⇨ infections, aging, disease

- Polyunsaturated oils (bean, seed), atmospheric radiation, pollution increases free radicals (aging)
- Deficiency ⇨ night blindness, dry skin, fatigue, insomnia, skin disorders
- Excess (>100,000 IU)/ day) in the extreme can damage the liver, spleen, sex organs, skin

Food, herbs
- Fish liver oils, liver
- Dark leafy greens (kale, collards, dandelion, beet)
- Carrots (carotenoids, converted by liver ⇨ Vitamin A)
- Spinach, yellow squash, sweet potatoes
- Parsley, spirulina, kelp, peaches, apricots
- Alfalfa, burdock, cayenne pepper, horsetail, sage

B COMPLEX

a) Protein digestion, eyes, skin, hair
b) Nerves, brain, liver, mouth
c) Deficiency of one generally indicates deficiency of all

1. **Vitamin B1** (Thiamine)
- Hydrochloric acid, carbohydrate metabolism
- Blood, circulation, brain
- Deficiency ⇨ fatigue, nervousness, edema, difficulty breathing, numbness, beriberi

Food, herbs
- Egg yolks, fish, poultry, Brewer's yeast
- Kelp, wheat germ, dried beans, most nuts
- Brown rice, fennel seed, peas, raisins
- Alfalfa, burdock, nettle, peppermint

2. **Vitamin B2** (Riboflavin)
- Carbohydrate, protein, fat metabolism
- Cellular respiration, red blood cells, antibodies
- Cataracts, pregnancy, dandruff
- Deficiency ⇨ mouth sores (corners), dermatitis, dizziness, insomnia, hair, vision loss

Food, herbs
- Meat, chicken, egg yolks, fish, cheese, milk, kelp
- Broccoli, leafy green vegetables, mushrooms
- Alfalfa, burdock, horsetail, peppermint, raspberry

3. **Vitamin B3** (Niacin, Nicotinic acid, Niacinamide)
- Increases carbohydrate, protein, fat metabolism
- Circulation, lowers cholesterol, nervous system
- Causes *flushing, itching* (20 minutes +/-) when taken on empty stomach, less when in middle of meal. Flush free does not work as well
- Deficiency ⇨ diarrhea, indigestion, no appetite, low blood sugar, fatigue, muscular weakness, dizziness, insomnia, pellagra, canker sores
- Avoid: pregnant, diabetic, glaucoma, gout, liver disease, peptic ulcer

Food, herbs
- Fish, eggs, cheese, Brewer's yeast
- Broccoli, carrots, tomatoes, wheat germ, kelp
- Alfalfa, burdock, horsetail, peppermint, raspberry

4. **Vitamin B5** (Pantothenic Acid)
- Converts protein, fat, carbohydrates ⇨
- Energy, hormones, antibodies, anti-stress
- Deficiency ⇨ headaches, tingling (hands)

Food
- Beef, eggs, nuts, fresh vegetables
- Brewer's yeast

5. **Vitamin B6** (Pyridoxine)
- Red blood cells, hydrochloric acid
- Absorption: Vitamin B12, protein, fat
- Sodium potassium balance, normal brain function
- Deficiency ⇨ headaches, nausea, anemia, gum inflammation, arthritis, dizziness, fatigue, acne

Food
- Meat, chicken, fish, eggs, walnuts, beans
- Brown rice, peas, spinach, Brewer's yeast, kelp

6. **Vitamin B12** (Cyanocobalamin)
- All animal: high B-12
- Carbohydrate, fat metabolism
- Red blood cells, sleep, fertility
- Myelin sheath: fatty covering of nerve axons (carry nerve impulses)
- Deficiency ⇨
- Malabsorption, indigestion, constipation
- Pernicious anemia, bone loss, chronic fatigue
- Depression, palpitations, tinnitus
- Severe energy loss, dizziness, shaking
- Symptoms do not appear right away

Food
- Red meat, chicken, turkey, fish, eggs, dairy
- Brewer's yeast, seaweed, soybeans

7. **Biotin**
- Carbohydrate, protein, fat metabolism
- Nerves, bone marrow, hair, skin
- Deficiency ⇨ anemia, high blood sugar, muscle pain, depression, hair loss, insomnia

Food
- Meat, poultry, egg yolks, milk
- Whole grains, soybeans, Brewer's yeast

8. **Choline**
- Brain, myelin sheath, nerve impulse transmission
- Hormones, liver, gall bladder function
- Increases lecithin, helps digests fat, cholesterol, reduce plaque, atherosclerosis, arteriosclerosis
- Deficiency ⇨ gastric ulcers, difficulty digesting fat

Food
- Meat, egg yolks, soybeans, whole grains, lecithin

9. **Inositol**
- Hair, increases lecithin, fat metabolism
- Reduces cholesterol, hardening of the arteries
- Deficiency ⇨ high cholesterol, arteriosclerosis

Food
- Meat, milk, Brewer's yeast, lecithin
- Whole grains, beans, vegetables, raisins

10. **Folate** (Folic acid)
- Brain food, red blood, white cells,
- Protein metabolism, energy production
- Pregnancy, fetal nerve cell formation
- Deficiency ⇨ anemia, fatigue, birth defects, gray hair, insomnia, forgetfulness

Food
- Beef, chicken, tuna, cheese, milk
- Beans, grains
- Dark leafy greens, root vegetables
- Brewer's yeast

11. **Para-Aminobenzoic Acid** (PABA)
- Sunburn, intestinal flora, assimilates B5
- Deficiency ⇨ fatigue, indigestion, nervousness, white skin patches, gray hair

Food
- Liver, kidney, whole grains, spinach, mushrooms

Vitamin C (Ascorbic Acid)
- Antioxidant (counters, detoxifies toxins), bruising
- Adrenals, immunity, blood, infection, cancer
- Reduces low-density lipids (bad cholesterol), heavy metals, blood pressure, arteriosclerosis
- Increases high-density lipids (good cholesterol)
- Best: buffered (minerals) + bioflavonoids
- 500mg: maximum absorbable dosage repeated every 4 hours (1 day) for common cold
- Smoking, alcohol, caffeine, drugs, stress deplete
- Deficiency ⇨ fatigue, bleeding gums, poor wound healing, low resistance, cold, flu, scurvy

Food, herbs
- Citrus fruits, green vegetables, kelp, Amla
- Alfalfa, fennel, horsetail, peppermint, raspberry

Vitamin P (Bioflavonoids)
- Vit C absorption, circulation
- Protects capillaries
- Deficiency ⇨ easily bruises, cataracts

Food
- Peppers, black currants, grapes, plums, prunes
- White skin beneath peels of citrus fruit

Vitamin D (several)
- **D2** (food)
- **D3**: sun's ultraviolet radiation, most common form, synthesized by skin via 20 min. per day
- Hormone, growth, development, absorption, utilization: calcium, phosphorous (bones, teeth)
- Deficiency ⇨ insomnia, osteoporosis, rickets

Food, herbs
- Fish liver oils, milk, butter, eggs, oatmeal
- Vegetable oil, nettles, horsetail, parsley

Vitamin E
- Antioxidant, moistening, healing (skin, burns)
- Improves circulation, clotting, reduces BP
- Deficiency ⇨ anemia, infertility, dysmenorrhea, miscarriage, nerve deterioration

Food, herbs
- Eggs, milk, beans, nuts, seeds, whole grains
- Cold pressed vegetable oils, wheat germ, kelp
- Alfalfa, dandelion, raspberry leaf, rose hips

Vitamin K
- Prothrombin (blood clotting), bones, glycogen
- Deficiency ⇨ bleeding

Food, herbs
- Egg yolks, yogurt, oatmeal
- Leafy green vegetables kelp
- Alfalfa, green tea, nettles

MINERALS

a) Acid, alkaline, nerves, bones, etc.
b) Contracting, on empty stomach ⇨ nausea

1. **Boron**
* Calcium, magnesium, phosphorous absorption
* Brain, bones, muscles
* Deficiency ⇨ Vitamin D deficiency

Food
* Nuts, whole grains, leafy greens, carrots, apples

2. **Calcium**
* Bones, teeth, nerves, gums, muscles, enzymes
* Heart (heartbeat, lowers cholesterol, blood pressure)
* Deficiency ⇨ muscle cramps, numbness (arms, legs), joint pain, rickets, tooth decay, brittle nails

Food, herbs
* Fish, dairy, almonds, sesame, flax seeds, seaweed
* Dark leafy greens, Brewer's yeast
* Alfalfa, chamomile, fennel, horsetail, nettle

3. **Chromium** (glucose tolerance factor: GTF)
* Picolinate: most absorbable form
* Glucose metabolism, blood sugar levels
* Protein, fat, cholesterol synthesis
* Avoid if insulin dependent
* Deficiency ⇨ fatigue, anxiety, blood sugar ⇩⇧

Food, herbs
* Meat, chicken, eggs, cheese,
* Whole grains, beans, wild yam
* Brewer's yeast, blackstrap molasses
* Horsetail, licorice, nettles, oat straw

4. **Copper**
* Hemoglobin, red blood cells
* Nerves, bones, joints, skin (coloring), hair

- <u>Deficiency</u> ⇨ anemia, baldness, osteoporosis, diarrhea, skin sores
- <u>Excess</u> ⇨ weakens the eyes

Food
- Fish, nuts, beans, barley, oats
- Broccoli, leafy greens, radishes
- Mushrooms, blackstrap molasses

5. **Germanium**
- Carries oxygen, oxygenates the cells
- Immunity, eliminate toxins, poisons

Food, herbs
- Milk, shitake mushrooms, broccoli
- Celery, onions, aloe vera, ginseng

6. **Iodine**
- Thyroid gland, anti-goiter, anti-septic
- Fat metabolism
- <u>Deficiency</u> ⇨ mental retardation in children, fatigue, hypothyroidism, weight gain
- <u>Excess</u> ⇨ swollen salivary glands, diarrhea, vomiting, metallic taste, mouth sores, reduced thyroxin (thyroid hormone)

Food
- Fish, dairy, sesame seeds
- Soybeans, lima beans
- Spinach, garlic, asparagus
- Kelp, iodized sea salt

7. **Iron**
- Largest mineral in red blood cells, hemoglobin (transports oxygen)
- <u>Deficiency</u> ⇨ anemia, pallor, fatigue, dizziness, nervousness, brittle hair, loss; fragile bones, deformed nails: spoon shaped, horizontal ridges
- <u>Excess</u> ⇨ free radicals, heart disease, cancer
- <u>Avoid</u> iron supplements unless diagnosed anemia

Food, herbs
- Meat, poultry, fish, eggs
- Brewer's yeast, kelp, sesame seeds
- Whole grains, green leafy vegetables
- Almonds, lima, azuki, kidney beans
- Pumpkin, peaches, pears, raisins, alfalfa
- Dong gui, fennel, horsetail, licorice, nettle

8. Magnesium
- Nerve, electrical impulses, enzymes, energy
- Prevents soft tissue calcification, stool softener
- Deficiency ⇨ weak muscles, heart disease (rapid heartbeat, hypertension, seizures), irritability, insomnia, diabetes

Food, herbs
- Meat, fish, dairy, eggs, whole grains, soybeans
- Green leafy vegetables, parsley apples, apricots
- Grapefruit, peaches, Brewer's yeast, kelp
- Alfalfa, cayenne, horsetail, licorice, nettle

9. Manganese
- Energy, bone growth, reproduction
- Cartilage and synovial fluid (lubricate joints)
- Nerves, mother's milk, protein, fat metabolism
- Deficiency (rare)

Food, herbs
- Egg yolks, whole grains, nuts, seeds, beans
- Seaweeds, green leafy vegetables, pineapple
- Alfalfa, dandelion, chamomile, horsetail, parsley

10. Phosphorous
- Heart, kidneys, bones, teeth, clotting, digestion
- Deficiency (rare)
- Excess ⇨ decreases calcium absorption

Food
- Poultry, eggs, fish, dairy, Brewer's yeast
- Whole grains, nuts, seeds, beans, seaweed
- Green leafy vegetables, pineapple, dried fruit

11. Potassium

- Diuretic, increases urination, eliminates sodium, helps maintain water balance, blood pressure
- Improves nutrient absorption, blood
- Tobacco, caffeine decreases absorption
- Deficiency ⇨ constipation, diarrhea, dry skin, thirst, insomnia, low blood pressure, muscular fatigue, salt retention, edema

Food
- Vegetables, fruit, whole grains

12. Selenium

- Antioxidant: inhibits oxidation of fat
- Heart, liver, pancreas, immune system
- Regulates thyroxin, thyroid (fat metabolism)
- Anti-tumor (lungs, colon, prostate)
- Deficiency ⇨ infection, exhaustion, poor growth high cholesterol, liver, pancreas dysfunction
- Excess ⇨ hair, tooth loss, brittle nails, pallor, arthritis, metallic taste, garlicky breath

Food, herbs
- Meat, chicken, dairy, Brewer's yeast, kelp
- Brazil nuts, whole grains, vegetables
- Alfalfa, fennel, horsetail, nettle, parsley

13. Silicon

- Bones, cartilage, nails, skin, hair, immunity
- Collagen (protein of connective tissues)
- Calcium absorption, osteoporosis
- Counters effects of aluminum
- Softens arteries, anti-aging, Alzheimer's
- Silicon levels decrease with age

Food, herbs
- Whole grains, soybeans, leafy greens, beets
- Alfalfa, horsetail and silica supplements

14. Sodium

- Blood pH (acid/ alkaline), water balance, nerves
- Muscles, dissolves solids, moves down (laxative)

- Daily requirement: 2,300 mg (1 tsp. table salt), 30 (celery, 1 medium stalk), 100 (6 oz. sirloin steak)
- Deficiency via low sodium diets, diuretics ⇨ cramps, headaches, dizziness
- Excess ⇨ edema, potassium deficiency, high blood pressure

Food
- Salt, seaweed, meat

15. Sulfur
- Protects, cleanses, disinfects blood, skin (harmful chemicals, poisons, bacteria, etc.)
- Counters radiation, supplements kidneys

Food, herbs
- Fish, eggs, beans, wheat germ, cabbage, onions
- Turnips, kale, horsetail, MSM (supplement)

16. Zinc
- Prostate, reproductive organs, immune system
- Bones, skin, taste, smell
- Deficiency ⇨ loss of smell, taste; hair loss, acne, fingernail deformation (thin, cracked, white spots), delayed sexual maturation, infertility, impotence, prostate disease, weak immunity

Food, herbs
- Meat, poultry, fish, egg yolks (avoid: swollen prostate)
- Pumpkin seeds, beans, sunflower seeds, whole grains
- Kelp, alfalfa, burdock, chamomile, fennel

ENZYMES

a) 20,000+ proteins produced by the body
- Catalyze, speed up biological, chemical reactions

b) Twelve major enzymes control
- Digestion, assimilation (carbohydrates, protein, fat)

Pancreatic enzymes digest carbohydrates, protein, fat. Too little protein ⇨ extreme ⇨ decreased enzyme production, which also decreases with age. Supplementation may be necessary. Hot spices increase digestion.

1. Digestive

a) Amylase (saliva, pancreatic, intestinal juices) ⇨ carbohydrates

b) Protease (stomach, pancreatic, intestinal juices) ⇨ protein

c) Lipase (stomach, pancreatic juices) ⇨ fat

2. Metabolic ⇨
- Cellular energy production, detoxification
- Construct nutrients into bodily tissues
- Heat sensitive, generally destroyed by cooking

Two:
a) SOD (super oxide dismutase): antioxidant
b) Catalase: breaks down hydrogen peroxide (metabolic waste, free radical), releases oxygen

Food
- Apples, bananas, mangos, papayas, pineapple
- Avocados, sprouts (very high)
- Alfalfa, cabbage, wheat, barley grass, sprouts

3. HERBS, EAST AND WEST

Plant medicine. Herbs (no protein, fat):
- Heat, cool, dry, air, moisten, purify, cleanse
- Move, hold, detoxify, antibacterial, antifungal
- Supplement, do not replace diet
- Generally powerless without corrective diet
- Generally safe, but can harm when misused
- May conflict with prescription drugs

There are only **five** herbs, categories, separated, defined according to overall **taste** and **energy**. (1) bitter: cooling, drying (2) astringent: cooling, drying, (3) sweet: cooling, moistening, (4) sour: heating, moistening, (5) pungent: heating, drying.

General use (+/- M.D.):
- With or after meals, temporary until better health
- Dosage (manufacturer's instructions, herb books)
- Temporary: 2x/ day, 6x/ week, 1- 2 weeks +/- or long-term, especially tonics, herbs (sweet taste)
- Best quality, strongest: **organic**, **raw herb** or **extract** (pure, no fiber), tinctures: non-alcohol, alcohol (place in boiled water, 5 min. eliminated) >>> freshly ground >> capsules >>> tablets (fillers)

Preparation: raw herbs
a) Roots, bark, tubers, berries: simmer 10 min.
b) Stems, leaves, flowers: infusion: soak 1 TB in 2C boiled water, cover, sit 15 min. = 3 servings
c) Seeds (whole): simmer (boil, low fire) 5 minutes

I. **Sour**: heating, moistening

1. **Amla** (amalaki) fruit (sour, cooling, sweet)
- Rejuvenative (blood, heart, eyes), anemia
- Premature greying, hair loss, weak spleen, liver
- Mental disorders, regulates blood sugar
- Cleanses mouth, intestines; hemorrhoids
- Anti-inflammatory/ acid (stomach): gastritis

- Nourishes bones, teeth; osteoporosis

2. **Hawthorn berry** (sour, heating, sweet)
- Increases digestion, weight; vasodilator
- Strengthens heart, circulation (coronary arteries)
- Reduces clots, cholesterol, arteriosclerosis, palpitations, insomnia; normalizes blood pressure
- Avoid: ulcers, colitis

II. **Pungent**: heating, drying, expanding
- Spices: hot (most), mild (cumin, coriander, fennel)
- Naturally thin the blood
- Carminative dispels gas, bloating
- Diaphoretic increases perspiration, dispels cold
- Expectorant eliminates mucus, phlegm
- Antibacterial, antifungal, antiviral, alkaline
- Aromatic smell: repels mosquitoes, ventilates LG
- Take during daytime. At night ⇨ insomnia
- Excess ⇨ perspiration, itching, dry, throbbing lips
- Avoid hot spices if thin, dry, pregnant, smoker, inflammation (GI tract, UB), bleeding, taking blood thinners.

1. **Basil** leaf (pungent, sweet, bitter)
- Boosts immunity, reduces fever
- Expectorant, relieves wheezing, congestion
- Opens heart, mind ⇨ love, compassion, clarity

2. **Black pepper** fruit (pungent, hot)
- Increases digestion, expectorant
- Destroys toxins (intestines), diuretic, edema

3. **Cardamom** seed (pungent, sweet)
- Settles stomach, vomiting, loss of taste
- Reduces mucus, coughing, bronchitis, asthma
- Neutralizes caffeine, digests dairy

4. **Cayenne pepper** fruit (pungent, hot)
- Stimulant (digestion, circulation)
- Diaphoretic (onset: cold, flu), reduces mucus
- Avoid: inflammation

5. **Cinnamon** bark (pungent, sweet, astringent)
- Strengthens heart, circulation, digestion
- Warms kidneys, pain reliever (muscles, toothache)
- Diaphoretic, expectorant, colds, flu

6. **Cloves** flower bud (pungent, hot)
- Dries the lungs, disinfects lymph glands
- Pain reliever, oil (toothache), detoxifies meat

7. **Coriander** seed (pungent, bitter): mild
- Stimulant, diuretic, diaphoretic, carminative
- Relieves burning urethra, cystitis (UTI)
- Allergies, hay fever, sore throat
- Diarrhea, dysentery, expels mercury
- Avoid: dry, airy, nerve tissue deficiency

8. **Fennel** seed (pungent, sweet): mild, calming
- Strengthens digestion, relieves gas, cramps
- Dissolves stones, uric acid, harmonizes urination
- Promotes menstruation, lactation, expectorant
- Opens chest, relieves wheezing, swollen breasts

9. **Fenugreek** seed (pungent, bitter, sweet)
- Stimulant, tonic, rejuvenative, aphrodisiac
- Gruel: Increase breast milk, hair
- Avoid: pregnancy, cause abortion, bleeding

10. **Garlic** bulb (pungent, sweet, salty)
- Anti-bacterial, viral, septic; stimulates immunity
- Fresh: promotes sweating (colds), opens the chest
- Detoxifies blood, lymph, clears parasites
- Stimulates bile, reduces liver congestion, jaundice, clots, tumors, varicose veins, phlebitis, arteriosclerosis, high blood pressure, edema
- Increases circulation, urination, sexual desire
- Dries mucus; too much ⇨ toxic blood, bleeding
- Avoid: hyperacidity, pregnancy, cancer

11. **Ginger** root (pungent, hot, sweet)
- Settles the stomach, moves obstructions (SI, LI)
- Analgesic, dissolves phlegm, clears cold
- Stimulates immunity, reduces infection

- Promotes menstruation, warms the body
- Relieves motion sickness, bloating

12. **Ginseng root: Siberian, Chinese, Korean** (pungent, bitter, sweet)
- Tonic, rejuvenative, revitalizes body mind
- Promotes weight gain, nerve growth, digestion
- Avoid: tumors, cancer, hypertension, inflammation

13. **Milk Thistle**
- Promotes bile flow, bowel movement
- Reduces liver congestion, fullness, toxicity
- Stops free radical formation, urinary stones
- Stimulates circulation, reduces depression, lethargy, coldness, depression via deficiency
- Moderates menstruation, menorrhagia

14. **Nutmeg** fruit (pungent, hot)
- Increases nutrient absorption (SI)
- Calms the mind (sleep), excess dulls

15. **Parsley** leaf (pungent, bitter)
- Increases digestion, nutrient absorption
- Promotes menstruation, relieves cramping
- Reduces edema, kidney, gall stones
- Avoid: inflammation: kidneys, sex organs

16. **Peppermint** leaf (pungent, sweet, cooling)
17. **Spearmint** leaf (pungent, sweet, cooler)
- Expectorant, opens up sinuses, relieves pain
- Settles stomach, clears gas, stops vomiting
- Increases bile, relieves breast, liver congestion
- Reduces inflammation, stops spasms, lactation

III. **Sweet**: cooling, moistening, relaxing
- Avoid: edema, excess mucus, phlegm, urination

1. **Elecampane** root (sweet, bitter, pungent)
- Strengthens, heals lungs, expectorant, emollient
- Asthma, bronchitis, pneumonia, anti-hiccough
- Avoid: overheated, hypertension

2. **Flax seed** (sweet, astringent, pungent)
- Hi protein, calcium strengthens bones, sex organs
- Emollient (softens, smooths), expectorant, laxative
- Strengthens, heals degenerated lungs
- Use: raw, ground or tea (1 TB, 1 C water, 10 min)

3. **Licorice** root (sweet, bitter)
- Increases digestion, weight, endocrine hormones
- Expectorant, moistens, cleanses, opens lungs
- Anti-inflammatory, cleanses lymph, glands
- Relieves muscle spasms, calms the mind
- Inhibits absorption of calcium, potassium
- Avoid: edema, hypertension, osteoporosis

4. **Marshmallow** root (sweet, cooling)
- Moistens: dry mouth, throat, laryngitis, thirst
- Gastroenteritis, colitis, cystitis, bronchitis
- Hyperacidity, breast lumps, mastitis, stones (UB)
- Helps heal chronic sores, necrotic tissue

5. **Saw palmetto berry** (sweet, oily, astringent)
- Increases digestion, nutrient absorption, strength
- Increases testosterone, potency, weight
- Insufficient breast milk, incontinence, infertility
- Underdeveloped (muscles, breasts, ovaries, testicles)
- Reduces swelling: prostate, ovary, uterus

6. **Valerian** rhizome (sweet, bitter, pungent)
- Increases heart chi, yang (energy), circulation
- Restores the nerves, relieves depression
- Circulates chi, relieves irritability, promotes rest
- Stimulates digestion, removes accumulations
- Strengthens eyes, benefits vision
- Clears nerve channels of wind (vata); grounding
- Too much dulls the mind

IV. **Bitter**: cooling, drying, contracting
- Stimulate taste receptors and vagus nerve ⇨ production: saliva, stomach acid, enzymes, bile
- Supports liver function (bile)
- Supports beneficial gut bacteria. Excess destroys.

- Digests protein, fat, cholesterol
- Anti-inflammatory/ bacterial/ viral/ fungal/ tumor
- Detoxes, thins the blood; diuretic, laxative
- General use: end of meal (except digestive bitters). Empty stomach ⇨ nausea
- Avoid: thin, dry, smoker, pregnant, weak

1. **Aloe vera** leaf (bitter, astringent, sweet)
- Tonifies liver, spleen, reduces tumors, parasites
- Regulates sugar, fat metabolism; laxative
- Obesity, swollen glands, venereal disease
- Avoid pregnancy, uterine bleeding, etc.

2. **Aloe gel** (bland, bit salty): external use
- Moistens dryness, relieves irritation
- Reduces inflammation, infection (skin)
- Tissue repair, stops bleeding, lactation

3. **American ginseng** root (bitter, sweet)
- Increases digestion, nutrient absorption, energy
- Improves immunity, moistens, strengthens lungs
- Relaxes the nerves, induces rest

3. **Ashwagandha** root (bitter, astringent, sweet)
- Rejuvenative: muscles, marrow, semen
- Weakness, anemia, sexual debility infertility,
- Old age, loss of memory, muscular energy
- Nervine, nerve exhaustion, sedative, insomnia
- MS, paralysis, emaciation (children)
- With milk, ghee or yogurt. Avoid: congestion

4. **Barberry** root (bitter, astringent)
- Stimulates digestion, absorption, destroys toxins
- Cleanses liver (jaundice), gall bladder, spleen
- Berberine: diabetes, regulates blood sugar

5. **Burdock** root (bitter, pungent, astringent)
- Cleanses blood, lymph glands, increases bile flow
- Reduces fever, infection, inflammation, tumors, stones, gout, eczema, psoriasis

6. **Chamomile** flower (bitter, sweet)
- Stimulates digestion, promotes menstruation
- Nervine (calming): oversensitivity, insomnia
- Inflammation (mouth, gums, throat)
- Migraines, conjunctivitis, tumors, colic
- Candidiasis, vertigo, tinnitus (loud), swelling

7. **Dandelion** root (bitter, sweet, cooling, pungent)
- Reduces infection, inflammation
- Breasts, mammary glands: swelling, sores, tumors, cysts; diabetes, constipation, edema
- Liver: cirrhosis, hepatitis, jaundice, gall stones

8. **Echinacea** root (bitter, cooling, pungent)
- Antibiotic, anti-tumor, detoxifies blood, lymph
- Immunity, cold, flu, increases white blood cells,
- Reduces infection, pus, fever, inflammation

9. **Gentian** root (bitter, astringent)
- Reduces swelling (liver, spleen), inflammation, infections, fever, hepatitis, venereal sores, BP
- Avoid if weak, nervous, muscle spasms

10. **Golden seal** root (bitter, astringent)
- Antibiotic, antiseptic, antibacterial, antiviral
- Detoxifies, cleanses blood, lymph, liver
- Reduces infection, inflammation (gastroenteritis, rashes, itching, measles, open sores, syphilis, hepatitis, jaundice, eczema), hyperacidity
- Varicose veins, tumors; promotes labor
- Berberine: diabetes, regulates blood sugar

11. **Gotu Kola** aquatic plant (bitter, sweet)
- Nervine, nervous disorders, epilepsy
- Balances right and left hemispheres of brain
- Increases intelligence, memory, longevity
- Hair loss, premature aging, senility
- Strengthens adrenal glands
- Blood purifier, venereal diseases
- Activates crown chakra (CH. 29)

12. **Green** (little caffeine), **black** (high) tea (bitter, sour)
- Antioxidant, burns fat, lowers cholesterol
- Regulates blood sugar, insulin, reduces clotting

13. **Guggul** resin (bitter, pungent, astringent, sweet)
- Reduces fat, toxins, tumors, necrotic tissue
- Clears the lungs, bronchitis
- Regulates menses, regenerates nerve tissue
- Arthritis, gout, diabetes, obesity, cystitis

14. **Horsetail** (bitter, sweet, cooling, pungent)
- Diuretic, blood cleanser, regulates minerals
- Strengthens, heals the bones, connective tissue
- Reduces stones, infection, enteritis, cystitis, nephritis, vaginitis, prostatitis, gonorrhea, edema

15. **Myrrh** resin (bitter, astringent)
- Simulates digestion, inhibits thyroid (hyper)
- Female reproductive system, cleanses uterus
- Relieves pain, swelling, heal sores, wounds
- Gingivitis, pyorrhea, prevents tooth decay
- Removes mucus damp: bronchitis, leucorrhea

16. **Skullcap** (bitter, sweet, astringent)
- Vasodilator: widens blood vessels
- Improves circulation, heart, relieves pain, tension
- Calms the nerves, spirit (exhaustion, depression)
- Reduces irritability, anger, jealousy, hatred
- Heart, kidney yin deficiency (CH. 5): palpitations, nervous unrest, insomnia, excessive dreaming

17. **Turmeric** tuber (bitter, astringent)
- Purifies, rebuilds blood: anemia, amenorrhea
- Antibiotic, strengthens digestion: protein
- Regulates LV, GB, diabetes, pancreas (berberine)
- Ligaments, poor circulation, skin disorders
- Avoid: pregnancy, jaundice, hepatitis,

18. **Yarrow** leaves, flower (bitter, astringent)
- Vitalizes blood, removes congestion
- Varicose veins, strengthens reproduction: female

19. **Yellow dock** root (bitter, astringent)
- Toxic blood, skin eruptions, swollen glands
- Hemorrhoids, glandular tumors, venereal disease

V. **Astringent**: cooling, drying, contracting
- Reduces bleeding, sweating, diarrhea, urination
- Anti-inflammatory, heals sores, wounds
- Excess ⇨ constipation, fatigue, dark skin
- Avoid if cold, dry, weak, pregnant

1. **Nettle** leaf (astringent, sweet)
- Nourishes blood, hair, expectorant
- Relieves coughing, wheezing, allergies, fatigue

2. **Red Raspberry** leaf (astringent, sweet)
- Reduces vomiting, morning sickness, diarrhea, leucorrhea, hemorrhage, prolapse, inflammation
- Harmonizes menstruation, promotes lactation
- Soothes mucus membranes, heartburn, ulcers

More information:
- **The Yoga of Herbs** Dr. David Frawley, O.M.D, Dr. Vasant Lad
- **Soma in Yoga and Ayurveda** Dr. David Frawley, O.M.D,
- **The Energetics of Western Herbs** Volumes I, II, Peter Holmes

Food Grade Chinese Herbs

Some herbs are edible. You do not, however have to eat the herbs, just cook, strain, and drink the broth. Start with small amounts. Most Asian groceries carry these herbs (botanical, Chinese, Mandarin names). Check sources: China may have questionable methods of soil fertilization. There are alternative sources if you choose.

(1) **Angelica sinesis** (Dang gui) builds, circulates blood, regulates menstruation. Cook small amount 10 minutes, in soups with meat, chicken or barely, azuki beans as a blood tonic. Contraindicated: pregnancy.

(2) **Dioscorea** (Shan yao), wild yam strengthens spleen, stomach, digestion, kidneys, lungs, treats bed-wetting, diarrhea, diabetes, good for infants. Ground dioscorea (1-3 pieces) into powder add to food. Cook 10 minutes.

(3) **Longan fruit (Long yan rue)** nourishes blood, heart, spleen, treats insomnia, dizziness, palpitations. Cook 5-10 minutes.

(4) **Lotus seeds** (Lian zi) build energy; nourish spleen, kidneys, treat incontinence, leaking (sperm, urine). Soak 6- 7 seeds overnight or ground into powder. Cook 30 minutes, until soft.

(5) **Lycii berries (Gou qi zi)** nourish blood, eyes, vision, reduce indigestion, diarrhea, anemia, nervousness.

(6) **Dried tangerine peels (Chen pi)** reduce phlegm, bloating, gas. Dry your own.

(7) **Black fungus (Hei mu erh)** nourishes blood, moistens LI (dry, constipation), lowers cholesterol. Contraindicated: yeast, pregnancy*. Many Asian women eat fungus, mushrooms regularly, rarely develop yeast infections. They also consume less dairy.

(8) **Black mushrooms (Xiang gu)** drain damp, clean, moisten LI (dry constipation), increase immunity. Contraindicated*. Cook 10 minutes.

More info: Beinfield, Harriet, L. Ac, Effrem Korngold, L. Ac. O.M.D., **Between Heaven and Earth, A Guide to Chinese Medicine**

4. TRADITIONAL CHINESE MEDICINE

Chinese Medicine (Traditional Chinese Medicine/ TCM): offshoot of Taoism, Buddhism:
1. **Yin, Yang**: dual energetic theory of matter
2. **Five elements**: qualities, energetic changes, manifestations of matter ⇨ affect body, mind
3. **Three treasures**:
- Jing (sexual essence, DNA)
- Qi (chi, energy): fundamental substance, life-force of the universe, yin, yang, all living things
- Shen (spirit mind)

Jing, chi: material foundation of the mind.

I. **Yin, yang**

Energy vibrates, expands (yang) and contracts (yin), moves fast, slow ⇨ five elements ⇨ heat, cool, solidify, move, hold, destroy the body, sun, earth, all matter.

Yin, yang: dual, complimentary yet antagonistic energetic opposites (+/-), **balance** of the body, all matter with one opposite always in excess ⇨ changes ⇨

Yang (male) ∇	⇩ ⇩	**Yin** (female) ∆
Ether, gas, fire	5 elements	Water, earth
Sun	Solar system	Earth, planets
Spring, summer	Seasons	Fall, winter
	Body	
Hot (active)	**98.6°F**	Cold (resting)
Anabolism	Metabolism	Catabolism
Building	Nutrients	Cleansing
Protein, fat		Water, minerals
Animal, beans, nuts	Food	Fruit, vegetables
Boil, bake	Preparation	Raw, juice
Acid (1- 6) –	pH **7.35- .45**	Alkaline (7- 14) +

Five elements:
- West: ether (space) ⇨ air (wind, spring) ⇨ fire ⇨ water ⇨ earth

- **China**: wood (spring) ⇨ fire (summer) ⇨ earth (late summer) ⇨ metal (fall) ⇨ water (winter) ⇨ five major organ systems ⇨ liver (wood), heart (summer), spleen (earth), metal (lungs), water (kidneys) ⇨ govern all structure function. More info: Qi (II. B).

II. **Three treasures**: govern all structure, function.

A. **Jing** (sexual essence): fundamental life-force, genetic blueprint via parents (ovum, sperm, DNA) ⇨ body's primary substance, new DNA, etc. ⇨

1. Governs growth, development, reproduction, aging, all structure, function, moistens

2. Stored in **left kidney** (kidney yin, essence) ⇨

3. Transformed by **right kidney** (gate of fire) ⇨
   - Marrow, brain, bones, spinal cord
   - Sex organs, hormones, head hair

4. Limited: one fuel tank (sperm, ovum)
   - **Fountain of youth**: strong bones, fertility, healing, memory, sleep lush hair, etc. when full
   - Onset of **old age**, physical, mental decline ⇨
   - Starts: men (late teens), women (early 20's)
   - Consumption varies: use, sex, climate, etc.

5. Deficient jing ⇨
   - Premature aging, fatigue, weakness, dryness
   - Thin, dry, sagging skin, wrinkles, fragile bones
   - Cold limbs, insomnia, infertility, impotence
   - Fear, declining mental function, dementia

6. The following consume jing excessively:
   a) Sex, orgasm (CH. 16), deficient protein, fat
   b) Chronic stress, insomnia, extreme climate

The more sex you have, the faster you age, dry, weaken, worse when starting young of after age 40.

Moderation is advised to conserve, use jing for health or spiritual development (CH. 29, 30) instead of sexual gratification. You cannot change past losses but can control, conserve, regain today for a better tomorrow.

B. **Qi** (life-force) within body: activates all function
- Fueled by jing, blood (nutrients), oxygen
- Flows within jing, blood, nerves, organs, etc.
- Depleted by poor diet, sex, drugs, insomnia, etc.

Five major organs/ systems govern jing, chi and shen. Each has favorite (growth) and non-favorite (destruction) foods, herbs, etc. More info: CH. 6- 16.

1. **Spleen** (yin), stomach (yang): digestion, blood

2. **Heart**, small intestine: blood, circulation, shen

3. **Lungs**, large intestine: air, respiration, blood cleansing, elimination

4. **Liver**, gall bladder: digestion, blood cleansing

5. **Kidneys**, urinary bladder: water, elimination, reproduction, blood cleansing

All have meridians (energetic pathways) used in acupuncture. More info: CH. 28 (Chi Gung).

Major forms of Qi:

1. **Original Qi** (sexual essence in form of chi)
- Dynamic motive force of all organ function
- Floats between the kidneys
- Foundation of yin and yang
- Transforms Gathering Qi into True Qi
- Transforms Food Qi into blood within heart

2. **Food Qi** (diet, nutrients)

3. **Gathering** chest, lung **Qi**: heart, throat (larynx, voice box), unites original chi, air and food qi ⇨

4. **Primary (True Qi)** ⇨
- **Nutritive Qi, blood**
- **Wei, defensive Qi** less refined floats between skin, muscles ⇨ opens, closes pores ⇨ protective shield: environmental cold, heat, dryness, wind, damp, regulates body temperature.

5. **Organ Qi**

a) **Transforms**
- Spleen chi transforms food into blood
- Heart chi transforms food, oxygen into blood
- Bladder chi transforms waste into urine

b) **Transports** in specific directions
- Stomach chi moves food, fluids down
- Lung chi descends moves fluids down ⇨ kidneys, urinary bladder, LI ⇨ urination, defecation
- Liver chi transports chi: all directions

c) **Raises**
- Spleen chi ascends, raises the organs

d) **Holds**
- Spleen chi holds, keeps blood, organs in place
- Lung chi holds perspiration
- Kidney, urinary bladder chi holds urine

e) **Heats**
- Kidney and spleen yang warm the body

f) **Protects** kills pathogens: bacteria, viruses, etc.

PATHOLOGIES:

1. **Qi deficiency** ⇨
- Hypofunction, fatigue, low resistance to infection
- Atony: lack of normal tone (muscle, urinary bladder)
- Spontaneous daytime sweating
- Depression, mental dullness

General causes:
- Chronic physical, mental stress, overwork
- Excessive sex, exercise, drugs, grief, worry
- Deficient blood, protein, fat, water, oxygen ⇨

2. **Qi Stagnation** ⇨
- Swelling (chest, abdomen), reflux
- Constipation, gas, tumors, pain, purple tongue
- Depression, mood swings, gloomy feeling
- Irritability, anger, frequent sighing

General causes:
- Deficiency: Qi, blood, jing, protein, fat
- Overeating, immobility, smoking, emotions, age
- Clogged intestines, arteries; tumors, illness ⇨

3. **Qi Rebellion** ⇨
- Qi moving in wrong, opposite direction.
- Pregnancy or food clog (ST) prevents ST Qi ⇨ ⇩
  SI ⇨ rebels ⇧ stomach, throat, mouth ⇨ reflux

4. **Sinking Qi** ⇨
- Heaviness, downward bearing sensation
- Incontinence (urine), spermatorrhea (leak sperm)
- Prolapse (rectum, uterus, ST)

General causes:
- Long-term chi deficiency (lack of holding)
- Chronic illness, excess cold (diet, climate)

Qi deficiency, stagnation and rebellion are generally simple (+ time) to cure via diet, herbs. Sinking Qi is more difficult, requiring greater time, discipline +/- M.D.

C. **Shen** (spirit mind)
- Higher nature, awareness, consciousnesses ⇨
- Spiritual and mental clarity, happiness, wisdom

5. AYURVEDA

Ayurveda (science of life) via Hinduism defines, treats health, disease physically, mentally, spiritually via diet, herbs, exercise, etc. via three gunas and three doshas.

A. **Three Gunas**:
- 3 fundamental qualities of nature ⇨ create, preserve, dissolve the body, all matter
- Via diet, herbs, exercise. etc. affect man/ woman physically, mentally, spiritually for better (spirit) or worse (rajas, tamas)

I. **Sattva**: spirit (Spirit), seed, light, intelligence
- Highest, elevating, "good" quality, harmonizes
- Raises consciousness, moves inward, upward
- Peace, love, cheerfulness, joy, devotion, faith
- Clarity, wisdom, truth, virtue, health, vitality

Foods, herbs
- Dairy (raw, unpasteurized > pasteurized)
- Organic seeds, nuts (almonds, walnuts, pecans)
- Grains (rice, wheat, oats), beans (mung, tofu)
- Vegetables (greens, sprouts, carrots, potatoes, yams, etc., raw, cooked), fruit (dates, figs)
- Sweet taste: maple syrup, fresh honey (< 6 mos. old), sugarcane: grounding, calming
- Ginger, cardamom, cinnamon, fennel, turmeric

II. **Rajas**: mind, fire, energy
- Activates, increases or decreases sattva, tamas
- Discomfort, turbulence, distress, conflict
- Selfish behavior, emotional fluctuations
- Passion, lust, avarice, imbalance, exhaustion

Food, herbs (stimulate, irritate nerves):
- Eggs, fish, fowl, lamb, excess spices
- Onions, garlic, radishes, mayonnaise, mustard
- Refined, concentrated sugars (all), white flour

- Hot, salted, pungent, sour, fermented foods, drinks (miso, sauerkraut, alcohol, etc.); coffee
- Small amounts do not decrease sattva

III. **Tamas**: body, earth, matter
- Material force, evil, dark, obscures truth
- Animal nature, degeneration, disease
- Addiction, gluttony, laziness, ignorance
- Loss of awareness, deception, anger, violence

Food, herbs (clog, dull, weaken):
- Beef, pork, fish, organs, excess animal (any)
- Fried foods, overeating, pasteurized dairy
- Excess sugar, bitter, astringent (dries nerves)
- Old, rancid, artificial, nutritionally worthless
- Alcohol, caffeine, sodas, energy drinks, drugs

B. **Three Doshas**: biological energies: combination of five elements (ether, air, fire, water, earth) ⇨ physical, psychological constitution

I. **Vata** (ether, air, wind): moves, "what blows"
- Primary biological force, motivating power
- Governs all movement, nerve impulses, circulation, breath, elimination, kapha, pitta
- Energizes mental function, brain, spine nerves
- Resides in empty spaces: head, joints, bones
- Motor organs: hands, speed, agility; speech
- Sense organs: skin, ears, touch; colon (gas)

D. Constitution
- Taller or shorter than average
- Thin, poor developed physique, bony frame
- Small head, forehead, shoulders, chest, arms, hands, feet, nails, thin nose, lips, low voice
- Skin: dull, dry, rough, cracked, wrinkled
- Dry hair, scalp +/- dandruff, split ends
- Teeth: crooked, poorly formed
- Physically active, tires easily, prone to injury
- Talkative, well-informed, intellectual, adaptable
- Nervous, superficial, indecisive, negative

E. Food, herbs (airy, drying)
- Beans (except mung, tofu), smoking, excess salt
- Flour, yeast, rice cakes, granola, coffee
- Raw, gaseous vegetables, mushrooms
- Most fruit especially dried; melons, cranberries
- Bitter, astringent herbs, laxatives, diuretics, etc.

F. Disease (excess vata, air, wind)
- Abdominal distention, gas, frequent belching
- Hiccups, constipation, anemia, fatigue, fear
- Anxiety, headaches, insomnia, restless dreams
- Arthritis, muscle spasms, shaking, tremors
- Neuralgia, sciatica, dizziness, epilepsy, paralysis
- Nervousness, confusion, depression, worry

G. Treatment: **hotter middle diet** (anti-vata)
- Building, moistening, heating, grounding
- 2x/ day
- **30% Protein, fat**: red meat, chicken, turkey, fish, eggs, dairy; nuts (almonds, walnuts, pecans, pine nuts, etc.), seeds (sesame) raw, ground
- **20% Grain** wheat, oats, rice, cous cous
- **40% Vegetables** cooked (+ sesame, avocado, olive, oil): onions, potatoes (sweet, yams, white), carrots, beets, parsley, avocado, radish, seaweed, turnips, green beans; chilies,
- **10% fruit**: avoid dried, melons, cranberries
- **Spices** all (except peppers) 3- 7/ meal
- **Sweeteners** all, except white sugar (diabetes)
- **Herbs** sweet (saw palmetto, marshmallow), sour
- **Beverages** water, lemon, limes, sour fruit, milk

II. **Pitta** (fire, water): transforms, "cooks"
- Fire in water: blood (98.6°F), bile, acid, enzymes
- Digestion, metabolism, intelligence, body T°
- Resides in small intestine, liver, blood, lymph, sweat, sebaceous glands, oily
- Skin (luster, complexion), eyes, feet

A. Constitution, personality
- Average height, medium build

- Pink or ruddy complexion, warm, moist, oily skin
- Forehead lines, freckles, acne, moles, fine hair
- Strong digestion, appetite, circulation, muscles
- High pitched voice, sharp memory, intelligent
- Angry, aggressive, domineering, self-righteous
- Perceptive, discriminating, courageous

B. Food, herbs (heating, drying, moistening)
- Sour, salty, pungent, sharp tastes
- Red meat, pork, fish, fried foods, alcohol
- Fermented (yogurt, pickles, sauerkraut)
- Ice cream, nuts, seeds, raw onions
- Hot spices, chili, black pepper, mustard
- Oil (except olive, coconut, sunflower, soy)
- Tomatoes (acidic), coffee, tea, ginseng

C. Disease (excess pitta)
- Inflammation, infection, profuse perspiration
- High fever, migraines, insomnia, mucus (+)
- Acidity, vomiting acid, bitter taste, bleeding
- Yellow feces (bile), foul body odor, anger
- Gastritis, ulcers, urinary tract infection
- Gall stones, hepatitis, cirrhosis, jaundice
- Acne, boils, hives, rashes, psoriasis, pus
- Cancer, high blood pressure, arteriosclerosis
- Dysmenorrhea, endometriosis, prostatitis

D. Treatment: **colder middle diet #1** (anti-pitta)
- Less building, more sweet, watery, cold, drying
- 2- 3x/ day
- **25% Protein, fat**: milk, (low or no fat), cream, cheese (soft, unsalted), beans
- **25% Grain**: wheat berry, barley, quinoa, basmati rice, oats, granola
- **40% Vegetables**: 3-5/ meal: raw (lettuce, spinach, celery, cabbage, parsley, beets, carrots, sprouts) > cooked (cauliflower, green beans, broccoli, mushrooms, asparagus, Swiss chard), Avoid nightshades: tomatoes (high acid content) potatoes, eggplant, peppers

- **10% Fruit**: all, except dried (vata, air) or lemons, limes, bananas, grapefruit (worsen ulcers, UTI) in moderation, seasonal, do not mix
- **Beverages**: water (spring), 3- 4 glasses per day, tea: chamomile, green, raspberry leaf, dandelion
- **Spices** (mild): coriander, fennel, cumin, turmeric
- **Sweeteners**: all (except sugar) unless diabetic
- **Tastes, herbs**: sweet, bitter, astringent

III. **Kapha** (water, earth): sticks, solidifies, "holds"
- Governs form, substance, weight, stability
- Uro-genital, excretory organs, secretions, fluids
- Cushion, fluid solution where vata, pitta move
- Skin, mucus membranes, stomach, pancreas
- Chest, lungs, throat, head: where mucus collects
- Taste (tongue), smell (nose), lubricates

A. Constitution
- Shorter than normal; white, pale complexion
- Sturdy, well-developed frame, chest, shoulders
- Large head, forehead, wide eyes
- Thick eyebrows, nose, lips, hands, feet
- Abundant, oily, thick hair, thick, moist skin
- High appetite, heavy, hard to lose weight
- Friendly, jovial, sweet personality, content
- Positive, devoted, loving, sentimental, emotional
- Easily cries, temperamental, possessive

B. Food, herbs (moistening)
- Sweet, salty, sour, fermented (miso, pickles, sauerkraut, alcohol, etc.)
- Soft dairy, nuts, seeds, sweet potato, cucumber
- Fruit, juices, cold drinks, sodas, smoothies, etc.
- All sugar (except honey)

C. Disease (excess kapha)
- Stomach ⇨ indigestion, bloating, excessive saliva; nausea, appetite loss, heaviness, lassitude
- White discoloration: feces (loose), urine, skin
- Phlegm, cellulite, edema

- Lungs: congestion, asthma, bronchitis, pleurisy, cold, flu, difficulty breathing; mental dullness
- Obesity, diabetes, polyuria, sweet body odor
- Cholesterol, atherosclerosis, leucorrhea, yeast

D. Treatment: **colder middle diet #2** (anti-kapha)
- More warmth, fire, light, drying foods, herbs
- 2- 3x/ day
- **30% Protein, fat** beans: adzuki, soy, lima, lentils; soymilk > nuts, seeds, buttermilk, white meat chicken, turkey (condition, climate)
- **30% Grain** barley, quinoa, corn, millet, buckwheat dried, popped grains, rice cakes
- **40% Vegetables** lightly cooked, steamed broccoli, cabbage, celery, chilies, carrots, watercress, green beans, radish, beets; asparagus, turnips, raw sprouts
- **Spices** (all) 3- 7/meal: garlic, ginger, cardamom, black pepper, turmeric, cinnamon, cumin, etc.
- **Fruit** minimal: dried (all), cranberry, apple
- **Sweeteners** raw honey (astringent)
- **Herbs** bitter, astringent
- **Beverage's** dandelion, chicory root, ginger tea

Everyone's constitution is a mix of doshas: primary and secondary: v/p, v/k, p/k. Treat the primary more than the secondary. Severity of symptoms, climate, etc. determines diet and healing time.

Each dosha has a subtle, master form (vital essence): controls well-being, creativity, spiritual growth.

1. **Prana** (vata, air): cosmic life-force, vital energy ⇨
a) Material world
b) Body ⇨ brain, spine (CH. 29): highly concentrated
c) Feeds, invigorates ojas, tejas

d) Breathing exercises (CH. 27), sitting outdoors, fresh air, trees, staring up at sky (A.M., P.M.), stars (greatest prana): increase prana (CH. 29)
e) Meditation (CH. 30) controls prana (brain, spine)

2. **Ojas** (kapha, water, yin): vigor
a) Fundamental, vital essence, energy ⇨ physical, mental strength, vitality, vigor, patience, resilience, immunity, overall well-being, stability
b) Most refined, end-product of digestion/ food: provides deep nourishment
c) Essence of reproductive fluids, heats all structure
d) Rules prana, tejas
e) Deficiency ⇨ chronic disease, mysterious, hard to fight infections, hepatitis, AIDS, Epstein-Barr, premature aging, nervous disorders, etc.

The following increase
a) Dairy, organic whole grains, raw seeds, nuts (EFA) nourish brain tissue
b) Organic, fresh fruits, vegetables (greens, sprouts, roots, beets, carrots, potatoes), raw, cooked
c) Tonic herbs: amla, ashwagandha, ginseng

3. **Tejas** (pitta, fire, yang): inner fire
a) Digests air, impressions, thought
b) Increases will power, focus, insight
c) Meditation, silence, restricting speech increases

The following decrease all:
• Sex, drugs, hunger, devitalized food, overwork
• Excess mental stimulation, loud noises, smoking
• Anger, sorrow, worry, stress, anxiety, age

More information:
1. **Ayurvedic Healing** Dr. David Frawley, O.M.D.
2. **Ayurveda and the Mind**
3. **Soma in Yoga and Ayurveda**
4. **Yoga of Herbs** Dr. David Frawley, O.M.D., Dr. Vasant Lad

6. RESPIRATION

Body: 70% water, 65% oxygen. **Lungs** (spongey, watery, hollow, capillary, blood rich) expand and contract, inhale and exhale, control air, respiration, exchange of water-soluble gases:

1. **Oxygen** (O_2): vital nutrient, gas via sun, earth (green plants, trees) ⇨ nourishes, electrifies, protects, purifies, kills viruses, cancer. A few minutes without ⇨ cellular death, especially brain (30% of body's total), heart

2. **Carbon dioxide** (CO_2): poisonous metabolic, cellular waste, gas: protein, carbohydrates (grains, beans, fruit, vegetables, starch, sugar) ⇨

The lungs in Eastern medicine also control the skin, external immune system, large intestine, defecation.

A. **Respiration**

1. O_2 ⇨ inhaled ⇨ nose, mouth ⇨ throat (pharynx) ⇨ nasopharynx (passage way to nasal cavity) ⇨ larynx (voice box) ⇨ trachea (wind-pipe) ⇨
- Lungs ⇨ five lobes: 3 (right), 2 (left) ⇨ lobules ⇨ two bronchi (tubes) ⇨ bronchioles (smaller) ⇨ alveoli: sacs with capillaries (where oxygen absorption occurs) ⇨ venules ⇨ pulmonary vein ⇨
- Heart (top, left) ⇩ ⇨ all structures, cells

2. CO_2 ⇨ capillaries (blood) ⇨ venule ⇨ heart (right) ⇨ pulmonary artery ⇨ lungs, throat ⇨ exhaled

Mucus: water, mucin (sugar, protein), white blood cells via mucus membranes, glands ⇨
- Protects, filters, cleanses dust, smoke, etc.
- Too much or too little water, mucus decreases the exchange ⇨ oxygen deprivation, CO_2 poisoning

The following increase, decrease water, mucus.

1. Dairy: easily absorbable water-soluble **protein**,
    sugar (lactose), **water** ⇨ blood ⇨ lungs ⇨
*   Clear, white mucus, phlegm (thick mucus)

2. Digestion, 3 meals/ day ⇨ heats the abdomen.
    Heat rises, heats, dries lungs. Weak digestion
    cools the body, lungs ⇨ thickens fluids ⇨ mucus.

*   Excess water, juices, sodas, teas, etc. with or
    between meals dilute, cool, weaken digestion
    (CH. 7) ⇨ cools, moistens the lungs

3. Excess cold: climate (winter, a/c), food, drinks,
    ice water, etc. cools the throat, chest, lungs

*   Winter cold cools, thickens moisture (mist) in air
    ⇨ rain (clear) ⇨ snow (white), ice (clear, cloudy).
    Cold diet ⇨ clear, white mucus, phlegm.

4. Smoking, pollution, dries, poisons

5. Hot, dry climate, excessive talking dries, weakens

6. Home: green plants purify the air, take in carbon
    dioxide, create, let out oxygen.

B. **Perspiration**: receive, disperse refined fluids ⇨
    skin, hair

C. **Large intestine** (elimination)
*   Lungs expand, contract ⇨ moves diaphragm
    (muscular partition divides chest, abdomen) up, down
    ⇨ increases peristalsis (wavelike contractions of
    digestive tract muscles), moves food, stools down.
*   Lung chi descends, increases elimination.
    Breathing exercises: pregnancy, childbirth.

D. **External immune system**: skin, pores

- Open pores release heat, perspiration ⇨ cools the body but also allows entry of six environmental evils (heat, cold, dry, damp, wind, summer heat) if open too long via weakness, illness, exercise, etc.

- Closed pores retain energy, heat, protect, keep out six evils. Parents routinely tell children to cover head, neck, shoulders to shield, protect.

E. **Emotions**: healthy: courage; diseased: sadness, worry, melancholy. Sadness drains energy, fire.

F. Breathing exercises (CH. 27), regular exercise, fresh air, good diet strengthens

PATHOLOGIES (East, West)

I. **Lungs**, **Cold**, **Damp** via excess water, mucus, phlegm (clear, white) ⇨
- Coughing, wheezing, runny nose, sinusitis
- Shortness of breath, asthma, dislike lying down
- Decreased O_2 absorption ⇨ hypoxia, lethargy, sleep apnea, mental dullness, confusion, aphasia

General causes:

1. Cold climate (winter, a/c), in the extreme

2. Diet: excess fat, sugar, dairy, eggs, water, juice, smoothies, sodas, especially cold

Treatment: CMD #2
- Corn, mushrooms, radishes
- Carrot juice, tangerine juice (decongestant)
- Spices: peppermint: ginger, garlic, cardamom, oregano, fennel (relieves wheezing) dissolve mucus, phlegm; opens chest, lungs, sinuses
- Elecampane: expectorant, rejuvenative
- Mustard or cinnamon oil applied to chest
- +/- M.D.

Viruses: small non-living particles: nucleic acid, protein in animals ⇨ air ⇨ humans, lungs ⇨ bursts, kills cells, reproduces, releases new virus particles ⇨ spread, kill ⇨ infection, sickness (contagious)

Viruses thrive:
1. Stagnant fluids (water, mucus), cold climate
2. Weak immunity via poor health, low protein, fat, sedentary life-style, obesity, etc.

II. **Invasion of Lungs by Wind-Cold** (common, winter cold, less serious rhinovirus) ⇨
- Mucus (clear, white), body (98.6°F) ⇨ yellow, green
- Dry or wet cough, excessive perspiration
- Chest, sinus congestion, stuffed, runny nose
- Dry, itchy, sore throat, body aches
- Shortness of breath, headache, fever
- Stiff shoulders, neck, numbness, shaking

Viral infections, colds, flu ⇨

1. **Hypothalamus** (brain) increases body T° ⇨ 103°F ⇨ burns, kills some bacteria, viruses; increases circulation: blood, white blood cells

2. **Interferon**: cellular protein ⇨ viral immunity

3. **Immune system** (CH. 12) ⇨ white blood cells, antibodies: destroy, neutralize bacteria, viruses, poisons, etc.

Treatment: onset (day 1, 2):

1. Hot spicy (garlic, cayenne, black pepper, cardamom, cinnamon, etc.) vegetable soups, teas (peppermint) raise body temperature, **feed the fever** ⇨ increases sweating, opens the lungs, chest, eliminates mucus, phlegm, kills viruses.

2. Hot baths, exercise: same effect. Cover quickly after to avoid cold air ⇨ open pores ⇨ re-infect.

3. Golden seal, echinacea (bitter): antiviral, antibacterial, drains mucus, increases WBC

4. No cold foods, drinks ⇨ **starve the cold**

The common cold, if generally healthy, can cure: 1-2 days. Longer lasting colds generally indicate severe deficiency via diet (low protein, fat, etc.), sex, drugs, weak immunity, etc. may require an M.D., drugs.

Case history #19. friend (30's, athlete, Seattle, WA) at pool (Florida), parent's condominium, coughing every 5 min, said it was allergies. I said it was a **cold**. He needed hot foods. He held up his beer. I said I would make him a spicy, vegetable soup. He told me he did not like spices. Too bad. I went into his mother's kitchen, made him a dragon hot, spicy vegetable soup. He gobbled down two bowls. 20 minutes later: no cough.

III. **Wind-Heat**: summer cold ⇨
- Cough, stuffed or runny nose, yellow mucus
- Fever, sore throat, thirst, swollen tonsils

Treatment:
- Fruit, vegetable soup, golden seal, echinacea
- +/- M.D.

IV. **Flu** (influenza): mild ⇨ severe ⇨
- Cough, sore throat, swollen glands, sweating
- Fatigue, fever, muscle aches, headache, death
- COVID (CH. 20, Cold Flu)

Every year 10% (largely unvaccinated) of U.S. (40%+ vaccinated) catches the flu. The rest +/- do not.

Treatment: common cold recommendations +
- Tea: licorice (cleanse lymph, glands), cardamom, dried ginger (¼ tsp. each): anti-flu, swollen glands
- Sage: sore throat, laryngitis, swollen glands
- Bitters: turmeric, yellow dock, dandelion root, golden seal root, wild cherry bark
- +/- M.D.

Every year 10% (largely unvaccinated) of U.S. (40%+ vaccinated) catches the flu. The rest +/- do not.

The majority who suffered COVID, hospitalization, ventilators or died: age 65+: **obese** (excess fat, mucus, clogged lungs) = 35% Americans (1/6 children).

Major outbreaks occurred: meat processing plants.

Flu vaccine: generally safe, efficacious, strain specific, requires yearly, bi-annual immunization +/- booster shots for each strain: regular, COVID, etc.

1. Short-term answer, antibody (4 mos.), but fails to exercise, strengthen immune system, unlike occasional sicknesses which does, just as exercise strengthens bones, muscles, locomotion.

2. Does not change major cause of weak immunity: poor diet. Waiting for vaccines is a risky bet.

Not everyone who is exposed gets sick. The young, lean or physically active: hotter, stronger immunity, greater resistance, quicker healing.

Case history #12. I (73) lacto- vegetarian +/- vegan, spice, etc. since age 51. Last 46 years: no flu shots, colds, flus, fever but occasional coughs, sore throats cured 1- 2 days: vegetable soup, spices, herbs.

V. **Lung-Chi Deficiency** ⇨
*   Shortness of breath, cough, tires easily
*   Daytime sweating, weak voice
*   Bright white complexion
*   Dislikes, propensity to catch colds

General causes:

1. Genetic weakness via parents

2. Exterior attack: wind-cold

VI. **Lung-Dryness** ⇨
* Cough, dry mouth, throat, hoarse voice, thirst

General causes:
* Smoking, hot, dry climate
* Stomach yin deficiency via irregular diet, meal times, eating late at night, worrying while eating
* Too little protein, fat, excess spices

Treatment:
* TCM: white foods (milk, tofu, white radish, turnips) nourish, cool, moisten
* Smokers: peppermint tea, honey, slippery elm: tea, lozenges, drinking water after smoking +/- occasional coconut oil gargling (do not swallow), help cool, moisten, cleanse the mouth, throat

Case history #18. I (60's): dry cough, lips for five days, until I figured my vegan diet (low protein, fat), coffee, hot spices were too drying. I switched to CMD #1, dairy, reduced coffee, spices, etc. It took 2 days to cure.

VII. **Lung-Damp Heat** ⇨
* Yellow, green mucus, phlegm
* Cough (bark), bronchitis, bloody sputum
* Swollen glands, infection

General causes:
* Bacterial, viral infection
* Diet: red meat, pork, chicken, turkey, fish, eggs, whole dairy, fried foods, fermented foods ⇨

Treatment: CMD #2
* Radishes, turnips, elecampane, wild cherry bark
* Spices: fennel, coriander, turmeric, ginger
* Peppermint, camphor oil: inhale through nose
* +/- M.D.

VIII. **Tumors**, **cancer** (lungs, throat)

General causes:

1. Diet: excess protein, saturated fat, cholesterol ⇨ tumors ⇨ benign ⇨ can deteriorate ⇨ cancer

2. Smoking, vaping: tobacco (100+ chemicals, tar, nicotine), marijuana dries hardens lung tissues ⇨ **tumors** ⇨ extreme ⇨ DNA damage, lung cell mutations, cancer (lungs, breasts, mouth, throat, stomach), periodontal disease, addiction, death.
- More info: CH. 9 (Circulation)

Treatment: CMD (low or no fat dairy) #1, 2
- Organic raw red beets, lettuce, celery, greens: nitrates, nitric oxide, dilates vessels, increases circulation, oxygen, tumor inhibiting, anti-cancer; Use: 1 C organic (raw, or juice), 1- 2x/ day; contains oxalic acid (avoid: stones)
- Flax seeds: degenerative lung tissue
- Marshmallow, selenium, fresh air (trees, forest)
- +/- M.D.

30 years of daily smoking, pack(s)/ day (not advised) can be cleansed via cessation of smoking (20+ yrs.):

Case history #20. customer, John (80's) only bought selenium and lecithin. One day, I asked him why? He told me, a little irritated, that he had just returned from **Hollywood Presbyterian Hospital** for biannual checkup. His **pulmonary** doctor (30's) examined his x-rays, saw nothing, and said that **John** had probably **never smoked** a cigarette in his life. John laughed and told the doctor that he had been a **heavy-duty smoker** for 40 years, two packs/ day, but **quit 20 years** ago. The doctor did not believe him. John handed him his business card, told him to call his secretary (40+ yrs.) for verification. The doctor called in the head pulmonary doctor (60+), who said he could spot a casual smoker, one cigarette a day. He looked at the x-rays and said "beyond a doubt" that **John had never smoked in his life**, which made him angry. John then told me that 60 years ago, his doctor had warned him to give up smoking and alcohol ⇨ cancer and heart disease.

John refused, told his doctor that he liked smoking and drinking and was not going to quit. His doctor (grew up on farm, raised horses) advised selenium (horses, lungs) and lecithin (heart), which may or may not had helped clean his lungs, unlike 20 years no smoking and daily blood flow, head to toe, 1,000+ times/ day, which nourishes and cleanses the lungs, all tissues, nerves, glands, organs etc. This is no way advocates smoking.

IX. Weak kidneys (CH. 16) shorten the breath

X. Emotions
• Sadness, crying, depressing people, movies ⇨
• Drain, weaken the lungs

Treatment:
• Inspirational, funny people, books
• Exercise, walking outdoors (trees)
• Avoid depressing books, movies, people

"For the sake of one's vitality, one must not talk (form of chi, energy) too much." **YOJOKUN** page 45

7. DIGESTION

Digestion **transforms** (heats, purifies, reduces, liquefies, separates food ⇨ nutrients, fiber, poisons) and **transports** (moves food, nutrients, poisons, wastes down) via stomach (ST), spleen, pancreas, liver, small (SI), large intestine (LI), acid, enzymes, bacteria, bile ⇨

1. Absorbed (SI, LI capillaries) ⇨ **blood** ⇨ all structure, nerves, glands, organs, skin, etc.
2. Not absorbed poisons, waste ⇨ LI, rectum

The best diet can become the worst, poisons, waste is not fully digested. Cold foods, drinks (ice cream, salads, fruit, juices, water, etc.), overeating (per or between meals) reduce digestion, nutrient absorption and increase waste. Digestion rules blood, which affects the brain, thinking, concentration, memory, etc.

Three stages:

STAGE 1: food, fluids ⇨

A. **Mouth**, salivary glands ⇨ saliva (water, mucus, ptyalin/ alkaline enzyme) ⇨ liquefy, moisten, digests starch (carbohydrate) ⇩⇩

B. **Stomach** (ST, behind lower left rib cage), gastric glands, juices ⇨ hydrochloric acid (HCl), pepsin, lipase (alkaline enzymes) ⇨ digests animal protein
   • Sit, ferment (sour), dissolve ⇨ **chyme** ⇨
   • Pylorus (tube, end of ST) ⇩⇩

STAGE 2: greater digestion, nutrient absorption.

3. **Small intestine** 24' tube (3 sections):
   ⇩⇩

duodenum (left side) ⇒ ⇒ ⇒ ⇒ ⇒ ⇒ ⇩⇩
⇩⇩ ⇐ ⇐ ⇐ ⇐ ⇐ ⇐ ⇐ ⇐ jejunum (right)
ileum ⇒ ⇒ ⇒ ⇒ ⇒ ⇒ ⇒ ⇒ ⇒ ⇒ ⇒ ⇩⇩

1. **SI digestive fluids, enzymes** (alkaline): lactase (lactose: milk sugar), sucrase (sugar); bacteria (-)

2. **Pancreatic enzymes** (alkaline) ⇨ pancreatic duct ⇨ SI, digest carbohydrates (vegetables, fruit, grains, beans): protein, fat, starch, sugar

3. **Liver bile** (bile salts, bilirubin/ yellow pigment, bitter) ⇨ one pint/ day ⇨ gall bladder ⇨ SI ⇨

a) Emulsifies, breaks down fat droplets, cholesterol, lipoproteins ⇨ smaller particles ⇨ increases surface area for pancreatic enzymes, bile ⇨ greater digestion, nutrient absorption

b) Increases **peristalsis** (muscular contractions of SI, LI) ⇨ downward movement of food and stools

c) Binds with, helps eliminate toxins

Nutrients, poisons ⇨ SI (24'), **villi** (millions): finger, hair-like projections on the interior walls ⇨

1. Capillaries ⇨
   - Arterioles ⇨ arteries ⇨ heart (O2/ lungs) ⇨ all*
   - Venules ⇨ portal vein ⇨ liver ⇨ HT, all structure*

2. Lacteals (lymph channels absorb fat) ⇨ lymph nodes, capillaries ⇨ blood capillaries

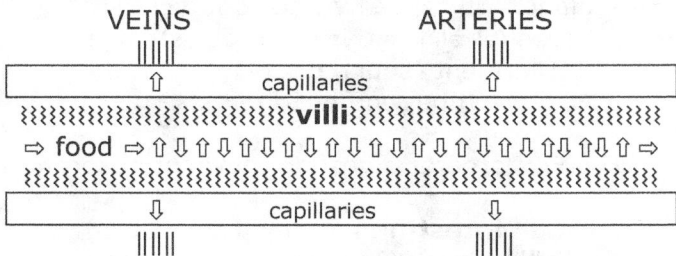

```
        VEINS                     ARTERIES
        |||||                      |||||
   ┌─────────────────────────────────────────┐
   │    ⇧        capillaries        ⇧        │
   └─────────────────────────────────────────┘
   §§§§§§§§§§§§§§§§§§§§§§§§§villi§§§§§§§§§§§§§§§§§§§§§§§§
   ⇨ food ⇨ ⇧⇩⇧⇩⇧⇩⇧⇩⇧⇩⇧⇩⇧⇩⇧⇩⇧⇩⇧⇩⇧⇧⇩⇧⇩⇧⇩ ⇨
   §§§§§§§§§§§§§§§§§§§§§§§§§§§§§§§§§§§§§§§§§§§§§§§§§§§§§§
   ┌─────────────────────────────────────────┐
   │    ⇩        capillaries        ⇩        │
   └─────────────────────────────────────────┘
        |||||                      |||||
```

STAGE 3: all foods, etc. not digested, absorbed ⇨

4. **Large intestine** 5' sac, tube (2½" diameter)

- Two sections (colon, rectum)

Colon (final digestion: bacteria, fermentation) ⇨
- Cecum (right lower abdomen, appendix) ⇧
- Ascending colon ⇨ Transverse ⇨ Descending ⇩

LI, digestive **bacteria** (gut flora) ⇨

a) Butyrate (fatty acid): strengthens lining of colon, reduces inflammation, prevents leakage of harmful substances into capillaries, blood.

b) Breaks down complex carbohydrates (grains, beans, nuts, seeds, vegetables, etc.), fibers ⇨

- Refined nutrients, air (Ayurveda) ⇨ blood ⇨ brain, glands, bones, immune, nervous system.

- Less refined ⇨ body fluids: tears, sweat, mucus, synovial, saliva moistens ⇨ mouth, skin, muscles, joints, spine, orifices (eyes, nose, ears).

c) Prebiotics: fiber (oats, beans, apples, bananas, raisins, avocados) ⇨ ferment in LI ⇨ beneficial gut bacteria

d) Probiotics: live bacteria, yeast via fermented foods (yogurt, kefir, kombucha, sauerkraut, miso, tempeh, etc.)

e) Bitter herbs (except turmeric), laxatives, coffee (excess), antibiotics, overeating destroy intestinal flora.

All food, nutrients, poisons not digested, absorbed ⇨ waste, poisons ⇨ **rectum** (8″) ⇨ stools, eliminated

TCM: spleen (chi, yang)/ pancreas governs digestion, stomach fire. Cold foods, drinks weaken spleen yang, digestion. All fire (yang) is governed by kidney yang, which is weakened by excessive sex, old age (CH. 16).

PATHOLOGIES:
- **>**= greater than, **<**= lesser than

A. Dietary

1. **Deficient protein**, **fat** (animal, plant), **eating too little** (⇨ lesser acids, enzymes), irregular meals, overeating, cold foods, drinks ⇨
- Weak stomach, liver, less bile (downward movement) ⇨ bloating, gas

Treatment: Hotter middle diet
- Chicken, turkey, nuts
- Rice (brown, basmati), wheat, spices
- Sweet, yellow, orange foods (millet, carrots, hard squash, etc.), rice: nourish spleen, digestion

2. **Excess cold** foods, drinks: salads, fruit, water, etc. ⇨ dilute weaken acid, enzymes ⇨

a) Stomach ⇨
- Bloating, gas, loose stools, tiredness (A.M.)
- Discomfort (ST area), better after eating

b) Small intestine ⇨
- Abdominal bloating, pain relieved by farting
- Malabsorption, pain in testes, worms (CH. 26)

Treatment: cooked foods, spices

Case history #21. Woman: 40, dairy, salads, juices, cold drinks ⇨ **stomach flu** (virus) ⇨ bloating, fever, loose stools. I made her a hot, spicy vegetable soup. She had 3 servings, sweated profusely, was cured next day.

3. **Excess protein, hot, greasy, sour** (sauerkraut, pickles, wine, dairy), **acidic foods, alcohol** ⇨

a) Stomach or phlegm fire ⇨
- Hyperacidity, thirst, desire for cold drinks
- Constant hunger, nausea, vomiting (sour taste)

- Stomach ulcer (lesion) ⇨ loss of appetite, pain, nausea, vomiting (blood), black stools (blood)

b) SI ⇨ duodenal ulcer, red stools (blood)
c) Pancreas ⇨ pancreatitis (CH. 24), tumors, cancer (CH. 20)
d) Liver, gall bladder disease (CH. 10) ⇨ insufficient bile flow bloating, pain, insomnia (11 P.M. 3 A.M.)

Treatment:
- CMD #1 (stomach), CMD #2 (phlegm)
- CMD #1, 2 (LV, GB), bitter herbs (milk thistle)
- Ulcers (CH. 26): bland diet, milk, ghee, whole grains mung bean sprouts, alfalfa, amla
- +/- M.D.

4. **Overeating, meals to close** (< 4 hrs. apart) ⇨

a) Clogs stomach, small intestine ⇨ reduces, mixing of food, acid, enzymes, etc. ⇨
- Bloating, excess fermentation, acidity, reflux
- Belching, halitosis (foul or sour breath), nausea
- Increased waste, poisons, malabsorption
- Heartburn (GERD): via clogged stomach/ pylorus ⇨ backflow of HCL ⇧ esophagus ⇨ burning, stabbing pain in chest below sternum
- High blood pressure via excess weight, increased retention of fluids ⇨ increase blood volume ⇨ increases blood pressure.

Treatment:
- Smaller meals, fasting: 6 P.M. - breakfast
- Vegetables: raw > cooked; heartburn: CH. 22

5. **Excess flour** (cookies, pretzels, chips, crackers, bread), nut butters, chocolate, candy; macaroni, cheese, cheese steak, pizza ⇨
- Paste, harden (SI, LI) ⇨ pain, bloating, gas, reflux, nausea, malabsorption, pasty stools
- Excess waste, weight in LI pushes down on urinary bladder ⇨ urgency to urinate

Treatment: weeks, months, depending on severity
- Fruit (especially for breakfast), vegetables (raw > cooked), water +++. Avoid coffee (drying)
- Smaller meals, less fat, flour, junk
- The less you eat, the more you digest, burn, lose weight.

6. Obesity, narrow, clogged SI, LI (protein, fat, flour, sugar), liver, gall bladder congestion (decreased bile) ⇨ painful bloating, gas, acidity, constipation, insomnia (11 P.M. ⇨ 3 A.M.)

Treatment: CMD #1, 2
- Vegetables (raw, cooked), fruit, juices, water
- Bitter herbs (laxative, stimulate bile): milk thistle, dandelion, burdock root, skullcap (insomnia)

7. **Poor food combining**:
a) Dairy + sour fruit, meat, fish (red, white)
b) Grain, bread, cookies, chips + fruit, sugar or meat
c) Beans + fruit, juice or sugar ⇨
- Bloating, gas, acidity, heartburn, malabsorption

8. **Taste** (Ayurveda): all food is digested, absorbed according to taste (6). Correct order increases:

Beginning of meal:

a) **Sweet** taste: fruit, sugar, desserts eaten digested first, beginning of meal. At end or between ⇨ gas, bloating, acidity. Most food (protein, fat, carbohydrates): sweet (main, major taste).

Middle:

b) **Sweet, salty** (meat, chicken, turkey, fish, eggs, cheese, nuts, etc.) digested ⇨ **stomach**

c) **Sour** (fermented foods) ⇨ **small intestine**
- Relish, pickles, sauerkraut, yogurt

d) **Pungent** (spices) ⇨ **large intestine**
* #1, 2, 3 + cooked vegetables +/- grain

End:

e) **Bitter** vegetables (lettuce, salad greens), herbs help produce stool, increase digestion in liver.
f) **Astringent** vegetables (greens), herbs

Astringent or bitter herbs (except small amounts), coffee (bitter), especially in A.M., empty stomach or beginning of meal, weaken digestion.

9. **Eating times**

TCM: digestion (ST, SI): strongest, highly charged:
* 7 A.M. – 3 P.M. via sun, activity, upright posture ⇨ better digestion (protein, fat, overeating), mixing acid, enzymes, downward movement: SI, LI (29') ⇨ **6- 10 hours** to fully digest, absorb, move down

* **Building** foods (animal), nutrients (saturated fat, cholesterol >>> protein), largest meals: hardest, longest to digest, transport, generally **eaten early** (7A.M.- 3P.M.), begin/ middle of meal

* Eat like a king for breakfast, a queen (lesser) for lunch and pauper (least) for dinner.
* Regular eating times train, strengthen digestion. Irregular weakens.

* Overeating, late (7 P.M.) or meals too close (< 4 hours +/-), sitting, reclining or soon going (< 4 hours) to bed: harder, longer to digest.

* Eat while sitting, relax 20 min. after, then move around, stay upright (4+ hours) to better digest.

10. **Eating** while reading, watching TV or standing ⇨ directs blood away from digestion ⇨ brain or legs.

B.   Miscellaneous

1. **Age**. It takes energy to digest, Energy declines with age. The same large, close or late meals easily digested, moved down in youth, are now harder, clog, bloat. Supplements (+/-): digestive enzymes, HCl, bitter herbs.

2. **Emotions**. Excessive worry, pensiveness, anxiety, manic behavior ⇔ weak spleen, stomach, digestion.

5. **Mental function**: digestion separates pure (nutrients) from the impure (poisons). Ayurveda: Agni (digestive fire): good diet, strong digestion ⇨ strong, nutritious blood, brain, discernment.

•   Poor diet, overeating, multiple foods, ingredients, especially synthetic (preservatives, dyes, long list, unpronounceable names) per meal ⇨

•   Blood ⇨ brain ⇨ cloudy thinking, confusion. "Mixed food produces mixed thought."

•   Commands more blood to digest ⇨ deprives, drains blood from, weakens brain, thinking

•   Weak digestion increases poisons ⇨ blood

•   Excessive reading, TV clogs, weakens the brain.

"To lengthen thy life, lessen thy meals" Benjamin Franklin

8. BLOOD SUGAR

Blood sugar (glucose, simple sugar) via carbohydrates (sugar, starch) via fruit, vegetables, nuts, seeds, cane sugar, honey, maple syrup, etc. is the body's chief energy source, controlled by pancreas (digestive enzymes, hormones), liver, kidneys, pituitary gland.

- Correct diet, kinds, amounts ⇨ health
- Incorrect amounts, kinds ⇨ extreme ⇨ disease

1. **Raw, fresh, natural** sugars, fruit especially organic: best quality, high minerals, low acidity.
2. **Fruit** (fiber, nutrients slow sugar absorption). Juice without its pulp raises blood sugar quickly, is less healthy, nutritious, sweet
3. **Grain** (high fiber) absorbs slowly, gradually raises blood sugar
4. **Processed, synthetic, old**: lesser nutrition, greater acidity, leaches calcium (bones, teeth).

Pancreas (behind stomach): endocrine (hormones) and exocrine (digestive enzymes) gland control sugar

1. Endocrine (CH. 13) produces hormones (CH. 8) ⇨ blood ⇨ regulate blood sugar (glucose):

a) Insulin, pancreas stimulated (high blood sugar):
- Transports glucose ⇨ cells
- Excess glucose ⇨ liver ⇨converted into glycogen
- Turns glycogen (sugar) ⇨ fatty acids ⇨ stored in the skin (insulation, energy reserve)

b) Glucagon converts glycogen (liver) ⇨ glucose ⇨ bloodstream ⇨ raises blood sugar

2. Exocrine (CH. 7), digestive enzymes (sugar, etc.)

Kidneys (anti-diuretic hormone) filter the blood, remove poisons, excess water, glucose, etc. ⇨ urine ⇨ urination.

All blood (water, nutrients, sugar, etc.) ⇨ **liver.** ⇨ processed. Too much sugar, especially high fructose corn syrup, juice, honey, natural, artificially sweetened, processed foods, drinks, sodas ⇨ fat ⇨

1. Fatty, scarred liver

2. Triglycerides (also via excess fat, oil, CH. 2) ⇨
- Thicken, harden arterial walls ⇨ heart disease
- Inflammation of pancreas
- Insulin resistance (precursor to Type 2 Diabetes)
- Regular exercise helps reduce

3. Excessive uric acid

Glycemic index (GI) measures, ranks (0- 100) how quickly carbohydrate containing foods and dairy raise blood sugar after consumption.

Non-carbohydrate foods: meat, poultry, fish eggs, cheese, fats, oils, herbs, spices: zero glycemic index.

1. **Low GI** (0- 55) foods raise blood slowly
- Fruit: apples, berries, oranges, pears, bananas
- Vegetables (most)
- Grain: wheat, quinoa, brown rice, whole oats
- Beans: lentils, chickpeas, kidney beans
- Nut, seeds: almonds, cashew, peanuts,
- Dairy (lactose): low-fat milk, yogurt, cheese
- Generally beneficial to diabetics

2. **Medium GI** (56-69):
- Breakfast cereals, granola, oatmeal
- Potatoes (white, sweet)
- Basmati, brown rice, whole wheat pasta, corn
- Raisins, grapes, pineapple, kiwi, honey

3. **High GI** (70- 100): raises blood sugar quickly
- White bread, rice, pasta, watermelon
- Instant oatmeal, corn flakes, pancakes
- Processed snack foods

PATHOLOGIES:

I. **Hypoglycemia** (low blood sugar) ⇨
- Fatigue, headache, dizziness, sweating, nausea
- Palpitations, tremors, anxiety, confusion
- Swollen feet, constant hunger, craving for sweets
- Short temper, blurred vision, insomnia
- Lips (numb, tingling), nerve damage, coma

General causes:
1. Excess insulin via injection or excessive secretion
2. Deficient protein, fat, sugar; fasting
3. Drugs, glandular, kidney, pancreatic, liver, immune disorders, diabetes mellitus
4. Coffee on empty stomach ⇨ sudden spike in blood sugar ⇨ crash ⇨ low blood sugar

II. **Hyperglycemia** (high blood sugar) ⇨
- Hyperactivity, dry mouth, excessive urination
- Sweet odor: body, breath, urine
- Extreme thirst, hunger, loss of weight

Both (not severe): curable via diet, herbs (CH. 22).

III. **Diabetes mellitus**:

Metabolic, blood sugar disorder (high) via lack, or failure of insulin to transport glucose into cells, which instead collects in the blood. Ayurveda, Chinese Medicine: insulin and water disorder.

General symptoms:
- Hyperglycemia (high blood sugar)
- Fatigue, hunger (lack of usable energy/ glucose not entering cells), weight loss, confusion
- Excessive urine (sweet odor), urination, fluid loss ⇨ dehydration ⇨ thirst, dry mouth via excess blood sugar ⇨ overworks the kidneys, filter ⇨ draws more water ⇨ increases urine, urination.
- Slow-healing wounds, sores (sugar dissolves)
- Blurred vision, seeing dark spots (floaters)

- Frequent infections. Excess sugar feeds bacteria (urinary tract), yeast (genital, oral areas).
- Acanthosis nigricans (AN): dry, itchy skin, dark velvety skin patches, skin tags
- Diabetic neuropathy: damage (excess glucose) to peripheral nerves: feet, hands ⇨ numbness, cramps, burning, tingling pain, muscle weakness
- Brain fog, confusion, stupor

Two types:

1. **Type 1**: juvenile (genetic) or young adult
- Autoimmune disease: immune system destroys cells that produce insulin ⇨ hyperglycemia
- Requires insulin + diet, herbs

2. **Type 2**: **Adult onset**
- Pancreas: little or no insulin ⇨ high blood sugar
- Insulin resistance: body does use insulin properly

General causes (adult onset):

1. Obesity, kidney, pancreas, pituitary disease, etc.

2. Diet: excess sugar (long-term)
3. Diet: excess fat (saturated, cholesterol) ⇨ excess belly fat: abdominal organs ⇨ insulin resistance
- Curable via diet, herbs, depending on severity
- More info: CH. 21, Case history #31

Mind over matter: European medical journal: **schizophrenic** patient (multiple personalities). One personality medically diagnosed **diabetic**, needed daily insulin except when he reverted to another personality who was perfectly healthy, did not test positive for diabetes, require insulin. More info: (CH. 20, Cancer): boy who visualized, cured his brain tumor.

IV. **Diabetes insipidus**
- Uncommon via pituitary or kidney disorder ⇨
- Extreme thirst, excessive urination

9. CIRCULATION

The heart (muscle, pump, 43,000 nerves) expands and contracts, controls circulation of blood (carries oxygen, nutrients, poisons, etc.) via its vessels: capillaries (10 billion), arteries, veins to and from every cell.

Blood
- 55% plasma (92% water, 8% solids: proteins, etc.)
- 45% blood cells: red blood cells (hemoglobin/ iron carries oxygen), white blood cells, platelets (clot)
- Average adult: 1.3 gallons (5 quarts/liters)
- Complete circuit: head to toe: once every 90 sec.
- 120-day life-cycle

Heart (East): additional functions, relationships
1. Manifests in the face, complexion
2. Opens into the tongue: controls speech, talking, laughter, sense of taste
3. Houses the mind
4. Emotions: health (joy, peace). Excess joy ⇨ agitation, mania. Deficient joy ⇨ depression.

Heart (chest, left center between lungs) is divided in half, separated by a septum. Each side has two chambers: upper (atrium), lower (ventricle) ⇨

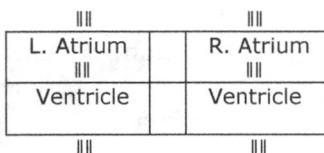

III		III	
L. Atrium III		R. Atrium III	
Ventricle		Ventricle	
III		III	

Vessels:

1. **Arteries**: 1 cm.- 2" diameter, thick walled, muscular, elastic, non-porous, expand (vasodilation) with each heartbeat, then recoil (vasoconstriction) ⇨ pushes blood through body. Arteries (do not clot) carry oxygen, nutrient rich blood. Exception pulmonary (carry poisons).

2. **Veins** (clot if punctured): 1 cm.- 2″ diameter, muscular, thinner (than arteries) wall, non-porous, can stretch and hold more blood than arteries, carry deoxygenated, poisonous blood. Exception: pulmonary vein carries O2.

3. **Capillaries** (10 billion microscopic, porous one-cell layer tubes) connect ⇨ arterioles (small arteries), venules (small veins) ⇨ arteries, veins.

*   Total length of vessels > 100,000 miles

Circulation: blood, oxygen, nutrients, poisons

1. **Oxygen** (O2) via lungs ⇨ capillaries ⇨ venules ⇨ pulmonary vein ⇨
*   Heart (top **left**) ⇨ atrium ⇨ ventricle ⇨ out ⇨
*   Aortic arteries ⇨ arteries ⇨ arterioles ⇨
*   Capillaries ⇨ most structures

2. **Nutrients** ⇨ small, large intestine ⇨ capillaries ⇨ arterioles (small arteries) ⇨ arteries (except pulmonary) ⇨ heart (top **left**) ⇨ #1

3. **Poisons**, **uric acid**, **ammonia**, etc. via diet, digestion, cells, tissues, organs, etc. ⇨ capillaries ⇨ venules ⇨ veins (except pulmonary) ⇨
*   Superior (upper body) or Inferior (lower) Vena Cava vein ⇨
*   Heart (top **right**) ⇨ atrium ⇨ ventricle ⇨ out ⇨
*   Aortic arteries ⇨ arteries ⇨ arterioles ⇨ capillaries ⇨ blood cleansing organs

4. **Carbon dioxide**: waste product of cellular respiration and digestion ⇨ capillaries ⇨ venule ⇨ veins ⇨ lungs ⇨ mouth, nose eliminated

Heartbeat (pulse): rhythmic beating of artery via pumping (HT). Adult: normal, resting rate: 60- 80 beats/minute. Young, healthy or physically fit: 50- 60 beats. Abnormal heartbeat (arrhythmia):

1. Tachycardia (heart rate > 100) via clogged arteries, excess calcium, sodium; low potassium (via caffeine, tobacco, lack of fruit, vegetables) ⇨ congestive heart failure, shock

2. Bradycardia low pulse rate (< 60) via excess potassium, low sodium ⇨ fatigue, dizziness

3. Poor muscle tone (heart, arteries) ⇨ irregular pulse

Blood pressure (BP): force of blood on arterial walls via pumping of the heart ⇨
- Contracts ⇨ beating: <u>systolic</u>, top # (yang, fire)
- Expands ⇨ relaxes between beats: diastolic (yin)

Normal BP: varies according to age, gender, etc.
1. Age 18- 39: female (<u>110</u>/68), male (<u>119</u>/70)
2. Age 40- 59: female (<u>122</u>/74, male (<u>124</u>/77)
3. Age 60+: female (<u>139</u>/68), male (<u>133</u>/68)
- Higher systolic # (varies) = high blood pressure
- Lower # (90/60, varies) = low blood pressure
- Daytime, stress, full bladder (high), night (lower)

Blood carries nutrients (protein, fat, minerals, etc.). Quality and quantity of nutrients positively and negatively affect the quality of the heart, vessels, blood, circulation. There are only two: building, cleansing.

I. **Building**: build, fuel, thicken, heat, hard, etc.

A. Nutrients (thick, sticky, hard)
- Protein (water-soluble). Excess ⇨ clot
- Saturated fat, cholesterol. Excess ⇨ plaque ⇨ atherosclerosis, arteriosclerosis
- Unsaturated fat: essential fatty acids (EFA) ⇨ HDL (high density lipoproteins) ⇨ breaks down fat, cholesterol. Excess EFA increases cholesterol.

B. Food
- Plant: nuts, seeds, beans: high protein, EFA, very low saturated fat; grains: low protein

- Animal: red meat (high protein, sat. fat, cholesterol) > chicken, turkey, hard cheese, butter >> fish (low saturated fat, cholesterol), eggs (high protein, cholesterol, low sat. fat) >> milk, yogurt (whole: high saturated fat, cholesterol > low or no fat) >

II. **Cleansing**: cool, thin, moisten, digest protein, fat, cholesterol, purify, cleanse, eliminate waste

A. Nutrients: water, minerals, enzymes, fiber
B. Food: fruit, vegetables

Correct diet (CH. 1) ⇨ health. Incorrect ⇨ disease.

PATHOLOGIES:

A. **Atherosclerosis** (thick, narrow, hard arteries via plaque build-up in inner lining) ⇨ decreases circulation, blood, especially to extremities.

Normal arteries (diameter) ⇨ maximum blood flow

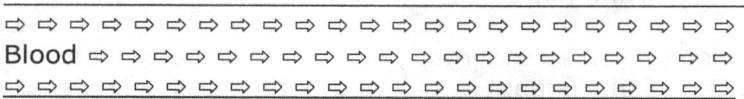

⇨ ⇨
Blood ⇨
⇨ ⇨

Abnormal, thick, narrow, bulging ⇨ lesser blood flow

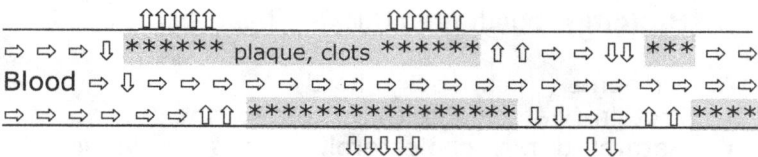

⇑⇑⇑⇑⇑   ⇑⇑⇑⇑⇑
⇨ ⇨ ⇨ ⇩ ****** plaque, clots ****** ⇑ ⇑ ⇨ ⇨ ⇩⇩ *** ⇨ ⇨
Blood ⇨ ⇩ ⇨
⇨ ⇨ ⇨ ⇨ ⇨ ⇨ ⇑⇑ **************** ⇩⇩ ⇨ ⇨ ⇑⇑ ****
⇩⇩⇩⇩⇩   ⇩⇩

General causes:

1. Diet: high protein, saturated fat, cholesterol (thick, sticky nutrients): red meat, pork, turkey, chicken, eggs, dairy (whole milk), fried foods ⇨
- Clots, high cholesterol, LDL ⇨ plaque ⇨ pastes, narrows, clogs, hardens (arteriosclerosis) ⇨

a) Coronary arteries (chest) ⇨
- High blood pressure (hypertension), cold sweats
- Nausea, red face, eyes; insomnia, loud voice

- Palpitations (sudden, rapid beating), tachycardia
- Angina: burning sensation, constriction, intense chest pain (left-side), extends down left arm

- Aneurism saclike widening or rupture of blood vessel (usually the aorta) via pooling of blood
- Seizure: convulsion: sudden involuntary, violent muscular contraction, pain, sweating
- Transient ischemic attack (TIA): mini-stroke generally via clot in neck artery: reduces blood to brain ⇨ drooping face (one side), slurred speech, dizziness, blurred, lost vision +/- blackout several days prior. There is no permanent brain damage. It generally resolves within 24 hours.

- Heart attack (myocardial infarction) death of area, cells of heart via blocked coronary artery ⇨ crushing pain (jaw, chest, left arm), shortness of breath, nose bleeds, dizziness, feinting

- Stroke (cerebrovascular accident) via blockage or hemorrhage of blood vessel (brain) ⇨ oxygen deprivation ⇨ kills heart, brain cells ⇨ inability to control motor functions ⇨ aphasia (difficulty speaking), paralysis, confusion, lasting brain damage, disability

b) Arteries (arms, legs) ⇨ peripheral artery disease, decreased circulation ⇨ pain, inflammation, numbness, shaking, stiffness, Plantar Fasciitis (CH. 24), Restless Leg (CH. 25)

c) Heart valve malfunctions: fatigue, chest pain, palpitations, shortness of breath, dizziness, swelling in ankles, feet: requires M.D.

d) Phlebitis: inflammation of vein (usually leg/ clot)

Treatment: CMD #1
- Beets, celery, lettuce, leafy greens (raw or juice): nitrates ⇨ dilate vessels, increase circulation, O_2
- Fruit, juices, water (+++), barley, oats
- Hawthorn berry (vasodilator) reduces palpitations, cholesterol, normalizes BP
- Garlic: improves circulation, reduces phlebitis
- Cayenne (helps revive heart after attack) + ginger (blood thinners) before, after angina. Avoid if thin, dry, or blood thinners. Excess ⇨ irritates heart.
- +/- M.D.

Case history #4. I (40's - 60's): high BP (150/110) + weight gain via overeating: cheese, pizza, ice cream, cookies, etc. I cured (weeks) each time via CMD #1, 2.

Case history #22. I (71, low fat vegan, occasional cheese) added ice cream, vegie burgers, chips, milk chocolate: high fat. Two weeks later ⇨ severe chest pain, insomnia. I stopped the ice cream, chocolate, etc. It took one week to cure. I went from one extreme (low fat) to another (high) ⇨ clogged coronary arteries.

2. Age, smoking (see F), diabetes, obesity, age

B. **Arteriosclerosis** (hardening/ plaque build-up) ⇨
- Loss of elasticity ⇨ decreased blood flow especially to extremities: head, arms, legs ⇨
- Forgetfulness, confusion, difficulty talking
- Headaches, limping, high blood pressure

General causes:

1. High protein, fat, cholesterol diet (A)

2. Processed, white flour: inorganic calcium ⇨ extreme ⇨ binds, dries, hardens arteries (arteriosclerosis)

3. Excess sugar, sat. fat, cholesterol, etc. (CH. 2) ⇨ triglycerides ⇨ thicken, harden arterial walls

4. Smoking (C:5), old age (dryness)

C. **High Blood Pressure** (hypertension)

General causes:

1. Atherosclerosis, arteriosclerosis

2. Overeating: processed foods (high in sodium ⇨ kidneys ⇨ water retention ⇨ increases blood volume), saturated fat, sugar ⇨ high BP)

3. Obesity (CH. 23): excess body fat, tissues require more blood (nutrient) to maintain ⇨ stresses, overworks heart ⇨ pumps faster ⇨ HBP

Treatment CMD #1, 2
- Raw or juice: beets, celery, lettuce, leafy greens
- Aloe gel, barberry, gotu kola
- +/- M.D.

4. Hyperglycemia (CH. 22)

5. Smoking, vaping (tobacco, marijuana) ⇨
- Carbon monoxide (marijuana: 3x > tobacco) ⇨ binds with hemoglobin (carries oxygen) ⇨ displaces, reduce oxygen supply ⇨ forces heart to beat faster, harder to pump, circulate more blood
- Artery damage, build-up of plaque ⇨ narrows (atherosclerosis) ⇨ decreases blood (O_2) ⇨ heart pumps faster to increase blood ⇨ higher BP
- Nicotine stimulates adrenal gland ⇨ hormones: epinephrine, norepinephrine ⇨ raises BP ⇨

6. Caffeine, alcohol, stimulant drugs

D. **Blood-Heat Attacking the Heart** ⇨
- High blood pressure, red face, red eyes, headache
- Nose bleeds, insomnia, loud voice, tachycardia
- Heat sensation, dizziness, anger, irritability

Dietary cause: excess hot, spicy, sour, salty foods:
- Chilis, pepper, mustard, tomatoes, raw onions
- Fermented foods: miso, soy sauce, sauerkraut, pickles, alcohol, wine, vinegar, fried foods

Treatment: CMD #1

E. **Low Blood Pressure**

General symptoms (TCM: heart-blood deficiency) ⇨
- Palpitations, poor memory, insomnia
- Dream-disturbed sleep, pale lips, hypoxemia
- Dull-pale complexion, dizziness, anxiety

General causes:
1. Dehydration (blood: 92% water), anemia
2. Medications, overactive vagus nerve
3. Smoking (D#3): damages heart ⇨ low diastolic rate, heartbeat, LBP
4. High blood pressure ⇨ extreme ⇨ low BP

5. Diet:
a) Long-term low protein, fat
b) Too many "cold" foods: seaweed, onions, celery, cucumbers, watermelon, red beans, green beans

Treatment: HMD (no red meat)
- Chicken, fish, eggs, milk, whole grains
- Ginger, cardamom, cinnamon, saffron
- Hawthorn berry, Arjuna, ashwagandha
- +/- M.D.

Blood pressure monitors are helpful. Blood pressure lowering medicines do not remove cause of HBP, LBP.

"For the heart's sake, one must not think too much. **YOJOKUN**, page 45

"As a man thinkest in his heart, so is he" Upanishads

"Learn to behave." Swami Sri Yukteswar

10. BLOOD CLEANSING

The body takes in toxins, poisonous or produces wastes via breath, diet, coffee, alcohol, smoking, drugs, pollution, etc. ⇨ **blood** ⇨ capillaries, veins, arteries, heart ⇨ most structures, including blood cleansing organs: **liver, kidneys, spleen, lungs** ⇨ purify, remove fat, poisons, viruses, allergens, etc.
- greater than (**>**), less than (**<**)

Liver (behind lower right rib cage), East and West ⇨

1. General (TCM): commands the body, troops: nerves, glands, organs, etc.
- Stores, filters, cleanses and distributes **blood** (oxygen, nutrients) ⇨
- Controls smooth flow of chi (blood, energy) to all structure

2. Cleanses the blood, removes:
- Saturated fat, cholesterol, bilirubin (bile/ yellow)
- Triglycerides, heavy metals, drug
- Metabolic wastes (uric acid, ammonia)
- Blood ⇨ kidneys ⇨ excreted (urine)

3. Transforms saturated fat ⇨ cholesterol. Saturated fat increases blood cholesterol by 25%.

4. Digestive enzymes: protein, fat, vitamins

5. Oxidizing enzymes: destroy, eliminate alcohol (poison). Alcohol reduces digestive enzymes, oxygen flow and destroys brain cells.

6. Bile (bile salts, bilirubin/ yellow pigment) ⇨ emulsifies ⇨ digests, breaks down, reduces fat droplets, cholesterol, lipoproteins ⇨ smaller particles ⇨ increases surface area for pancreatic enzymes, bile ⇨ greater digestion, absorption: small intestine (SI)

- Increases peristalsis: moves food, bowels down
- One pint/ day ⇨ hepatic (LV) duct ⇨ gall bladder ⇨ cystic duct ⇨ SI. Excess ⇨ feces (yellow).

7. Liver blood rules the eyes (vision, tears), sinews (tendons), nails, uterus

8. Greens (kale, lettuce, spirulina; barley, wheat grass): nourish, cool, moisten, cleanse, oxidize

9. Bitter herbs: stimulate bile, cool, cleanse, dry

10. Sour taste (hot, moist): stimulates liver, bile, benefits liver when deficient, thin, dry, cold; aggravates when overheated, clogged, fatty

11. Emotions: health (even-mindedness, patience), disease (anger, resentment, frustration, rage). Sad stories, books, movies, etc. drain anger.

PATHOLOGIES:

A. **Liver-Chi Stagnation** ⇨ swollen liver ⇨
- Abdominal distention, pain (below rib cage)
- Feeling of lump in throat, sighing, hiccough
- Distention of breast before period
- Melancholy, depression, moodiness

General cause: excessive frustration, repressed anger, resentment) trap energy, blood, heat in liver

Treatment: deep abdominal breathing, meditation

B. **Liver-Fire Blazing Upwards**
- Swollen liver, congested gall bladder
- Irritability, outbursts of anger, itching
- Red face, red eyes, temporal headache
- Thirst, bitter taste, nose bleeds (epistaxis)
- Tinnitus (loud), deafness, dizziness
- Red tongue, yellow coating
- Insomnia, dream-disturbed sleep

- Constipation, dry stools, dark yellow urine
- Painful, irregular periods, dark menstrual blood

C. **Damp-Heat in Liver**, **Gall Bladder**
- Fever, scanty, dark urine
- Nausea, vomiting, bitter taste
- Loss of appetite, jaundice
- Vaginal discharge, itching
- Rashes, stinky (groin), swelling of scrotum

Dietary cause: excess beef, lamb, chicken, turkey, fried, spicy, fermented, salty foods, drinks, alcohol

Treatment: CMD #2
- 2 meals/ day, spaced
- High fiber (whole grains, carrots, green beans, peas, tomatoes) helps reduce stones
- Mild spices (coriander, fennel, mint). Avoid hot.
- Barberry (swelling), golden seal, dandelion, aloe
- Milk Thistle, abdominal breathing
- +/- M.D.

D. **Gallstones**

1. Excess cholesterol, calcium salts, insufficient bile salts, lecithin or excess bile collecting in GB ⇨ crystalize ⇨
- Gallstones ⇨
2. Congest, obstruct GB, ducts ⇨ cholecystitis (inflammation of GB) ⇨
- Fever, nausea, vomiting (bitter), urine (brown)
- Pain: right side, upper abdomen or behind breastbone, mimics heart attack
- Backflow of bile ⇨ liver ⇨ blood ⇨ skin, eyes ⇨ yellow (jaundice, CH. 23); bloating, constipation,

Three kinds:

1. Cholesterol via animal, fried foods (B) ⇨
- Yellow, green or red, sharp, pointy, painful
- 75% of all gallstones

Treatment:
- High fiber (whole grains, carrots, green beans, peas, tomatoes) help prevent formation of stones
- Beets, celery, leafy greens (nitrates), avocados, lentils, apples stimulate liver, bile.
- More info: CH. 22, Gallstones

2. **Pigment** via excess bilirubin via break down of red blood cells, liver disorder, blood disease.

3. **Phlegm** via excess fat, sugar dairy, cold drinks ⇨
- Round, soft, whitish, generally painless

General facial symptoms: LV, GB congestion, heat
- Face: bright red ⇨ dark, purple
- Liver: vertical line between eyebrows
- GB: two, three vertical lines between eyebrows
- Lines, color ⇨ better (disappear ⇨ years) or worse

E. **Liver-Blood Deficiency**
- Dull, pale lips, complexion; brittle nails
- Wind: muscle spasms, tremors, shaking (head)
- Dizziness, blurred vision, see floaters (specks)
- Amenorrhea, scanty menstruation, cramps

General cause
- Diet: deficient protein, fat (animal > plant)

Treatment: HMD (avoid red meat)
- Cooked vegetables, spices, turmeric
- +/- M.D.

F. **Alcoholism** ⇨
- Liver dysfunction, indigestion, swelling
- Cirrhosis (CH. 20)

Treatment: diet, herbs, counseling, prayer: little or no value without cessation of alcohol

G. Hepatitis (CH. 22)

Kidneys: bean shaped, paired organs
- Lower back, left, right of spine
- Cleanses, filters the blood through millions of nephrons (renal tubules) ⇨

1. Remove water, nitrogenous wastes (uric acid, ammonia) ⇨ urea, urine ⇨ urinary bladder

2. Regulate minerals, electrolytes

3. Regulate pH: <u>acid (1- 6), alkaline (7- 14) balance</u>, prevents acidosis (protein, fat), alkalosis (fruit, vegetables, minerals)
- Normal blood pH: <u>7.35- 7.45</u> (slightly alkaline)
- < 7.35 ⇨ acidosis, disease
- > 7.45 ⇨ alkalosis, disease

PATHOLOGIES:
- CH. 11 (Elimination), CH. 16 (Reproduction)

Lungs (CH. 6, Respiration): blood cleansing

Spleen (CH. 12 (Immunity): lymph organ: removes old red blood cells

Skin (CH. 13): eliminates poisons via perspiration

11. ELIMINATION

The body eliminates dietary wastes, poisons, etc. via large intestine, kidneys, urinary bladder, lungs and skin.
- Retention of wastes, poisons ⇨ disease.

I. **Large Intestine** (LI)
- 5' tube, sac, 2½" diameter
- Receives food and drink from small intestine
- Descending stomach and lung chi aids defecation

Two sections:

1. Colon (4½'): digestion, absorption of nutrients
2. Rectum (8"): receives all food, nutrients not digested, absorbed ⇨ waste, poisons ⇨ stool

Normal, healthy stools
- Watery, semi-firm, temporarily float (+/- fiber) Relatively odorless, easy to eliminate in A.M.
- Indicates good digestion, high nutrient absorption
- 2- 3 meals/ day = 1- 3 eliminations/ day

Abnormal
- Stools: loose, dry, hard, smell, sink, do not float
- Diarrhea: frequent watery, loose +/- blood, mucus
- Constipation: infrequent, painful elimination

Quantity, quality and frequency of the stools are largely determined by diet, digestion, age and lifestyle.

1. Diet

a) Animal food (except soft dairy): hard to digest
- Thick, oily, hard, stinky stools, sink*

b) Flour: bread, cookies, pretzels, chips, etc. ⇨
- Pasty stools

c) Fruit, raw vegetables (fiber) ⇨ bulk, moisten, float

2. Digestion (CH. 7). Weak digestion ⇨ increases waste, stools

3. Age: Weak digestion, elimination ⇨ constipation

4. Exercise, breathing ⇨ expands, contracts lungs ⇨ moves diaphragm: muscular partition between chest, abdomen ⇨ up, down ⇨ massages LI ⇨ moves wastes down.
 • Inactivity ⇨ constipation

5. LI energetically active: 5- 7 A.M.
 • Early rising increases elimination
 • Sleeping late, sex, caffeine (A.M.) slows, weakens

PATHOLOGIES:

A. **Dry stools**, burning sensation, swelling in anus

General dietary causes:
 • Lamb, beef, alcohol, dried, broiled, baked meats

Treatment:
 • Eliminate animal, etc., increase fruit, vegetables

B. **Constipation** (CH. 20) ⇨
 • Abdominal bloating, pain, gas, weight gain

General causes:

1. Age, sedentary lifestyle

2. Excess bitter herbs (drying): laxatives, coffee

3. Deficient fruit, vegetables, water, fiber

4. Deficient protein, fat

5. Excess protein, fat, oil, flour

6. Weak digestion, downward moving energy

Treatment: CH. 20 (Constipation)

C. **Loose stools** via:
- Excess fluids, raw vegetables, fruit, sugar
- Bacterial infection, antibiotics, laxatives, enemas

Treatment: grain, cooked vegetables, spices
- +/- M.D.

D. **Diverticulosis**: abnormal, large pouch like sacs (diverticula) in LI muscles (common, age 50+) ⇨
- Few or no symptoms, occasional rectal bleeding
- Diverticulitis: inflammation, infection of abnormal sac (diverticulum) ⇨ cramping, bloating, tenderness (abdomen, left), nausea (relieved by evacuation), constipation, diarrhea +/- blood

E. **Tumors, cancer**

Dietary cause:
- Excess saturated fat, cholesterol, protein
- Red meat, pork, chicken, fried foods, butter, etc.
- Flour, sugar, overeating, sedentary lifestyle

Treatment: CH. 20 (Cancer)
- +/- M.D.

F. **Diarrhea** (CH. 21) ⇨
- Loose, watery stools, cramps
- Fatigue, dehydration, death

General causes:
- Excess greasy, hot, cold, oil, spoiled foods
- Poor food combining: milk + meat or fish
- IBS, Crohn's, drugs, antibiotics (cold)
- Contaminated foods, water: bacteria, parasites

Treatment:
- Cooked vegetables, spices, bitter herbs
- +/- M.D.

II. **Kidneys, Urinary Bladder** (UB)

Kidneys: bean shaped, paired organs in the lower back, on either side of the spine ⇨

1. Filter the blood, remove water, minerals, nitrogenous wastes (uric acid) ⇨ urine ⇨ ureters (thick-walled tubes, 12") ⇨ UB ⇨ urethra
- Kidney yang (CH. 16) thins the urine

2. Regulate minerals: sodium, potassium ⇨ control body fluids: intra, extra cellular.

a) **Sodium** stimulates kidneys, urination. Minimum daily requirement: 1,500- 2,300 mg. Too much ⇨ edema, high blood pressure.

b) **Potassium** (fruit, vegetables): natural diuretic, increases urination, reduces sodium.

PATHOLOGIES:

A. **Urinary tract infection** (UTI) ⇨
- Dark yellow, red (blood), painful, burning
- Cystitis (inflammation of urethra, ureter)

General dietary cause:
- Excess protein, fat, sugar, alcohol

Treatment: CMD #1, 2
- More info: UTI (CH. 26) includes cystitis

B. **Excessive urination** day, night (nocturia) ⇨
- Overworks, weakens kidneys, urinary bladder ⇨
- Incontinence, edema

General causes:

1. Excess fluids (water, juice, soda, beer, etc.). Eight glasses water/ day: beneficial if hot, dry, active or hot climate; harmful if weak, obese, excessive urination, perspiration, or cold climate.

2. Excess bitter herbs, diuretics, coffee stimulate, overwork, weaken the kidneys, UB ⇨ incontinence

3. Old age (decline in antidiuretic hormone) ⇨
- Incontinence: uncontrollable urination, nocturia

Treatment:
- Nutmeg, saw palmetto berry, lotus seeds
- +/- M.D.

4. Obesity, injury, Alzheimer's

C. **Urine: sweet odor** (hyperglycemia, diabetes)

D. **Kidney stones** ⇨
- Frequent urination (odorous, cloudy, pus, blood)
- Chills, fever, profuse sweating
- Pain radiating from groin, abdomen to upper back
- Urinary tract infection, dysuria (+ blood)
- Affects mostly white men 30-50 (high protein, fat)

General causes:
- Excess dietary calcium oxalate, uric acid, etc.
- More info: CH. 23

E. **Kidney yang deficiency** (CH. 16)
- Abundant, clear or clear scanty urination

F. **Kidney-Chi Not Firm** (CH. 16)
- Dribbling after urination, week stream

G. **Fear** in children via parents, siblings, etc. ⇨
- Bedwetting

H. **Resisting** urge to urinate, **holding** urine too long, weakens the kidneys, urinary bladder

I. **Kidney failure** via diet, sex, poisons, etc. ⇨
- Uremia ⇨ excess urea, nitrogenous wastes in blood ⇨ nausea, vomiting, lethargy, death
- Treatment: M.D.

I read a story about a sick young man (30's, weak kidney) who was told by his doctors (India) that he needed a **kidney transplant** or he would die. He then went to a yogi who told him (1) stop eating meat, chicken, fish (high uric acid weakens kidneys) and (2) eat more fruit, vegetables. His kidney healed. Everything changes.

III. **Lungs** (CH. 6) eliminate carbon dioxide.

12. IMMUNITY

Immune system (adaptive immunity) via cells, glands, lymph nodes, veins, capillaries, white blood cells (WBC), antibodies, etc. ⇨ destroy, eliminate many poisonous substances, bacteria, viruses, cancer, etc.

Viruses: non-living toxic air-borne particles via animals ⇨ humans ⇨ lungs ⇨ grows, bursts, kills the host cells, reproduces, releases new virus particles ⇨
1. Common cold (rhinovirus): less serious
2. Flu, COVID 19 (more serious) ⇨ swollen glands, tonsillitis, strep throat +/- death

Viruses, bacteria thrive in stagnant fluids (water, mucus). Higher body temperatures via hot diet (protein, fat, cooked foods, spices), digestion (acid, enzymes, 3 meals/ day), exercise and sunshine heat, dry, kill many bacteria, viruses. Colder body temperatures via cold diet, climate ⇨ thicken fluids ⇨ mucus.

Viral, bacterial infections ⇨

1. **Hypothalamus** (brain) increases body temperature (normal: 98.6°F) ⇨ 103°F ⇨
   - Kills some bacteria, viruses
   - Increases circulation, distribution of WBC

2. **Cells**: protein (interferon) ⇨ immunity to viruses

3. **Thymus, bone marrow** ⇨ white blood cells ⇨

a) Lymphocytes
   - **T cells**: cellular immunity (transplants)
   - **B cells** (anti-bacterial, fungal) ⇨ **antibodies** (proteins) ⇨ engulf, neutralize, destroy specific antigens, poisonous organisms, substances: microbial (bacteria, viruses) and non-microbial (pollen, eggs whites, non-compatible cells) ⇨

b) Leukocytes (antibacterial, fungal) ⇨

4. **Lymph system**

a) Lymph: thin fluid, 80% via liver, digestive organs, carries WBC ⇨

b) Lymph capillaries: microscopic tubes (most structures) ⇨ bathes, removes foreign substances, bacteria, viruses, etc. ⇨

c) Lymph veins ⇨

d) Lymph nodes, glands: neck, groin, tonsils, adenoids, armpits, spleen filter, kill, eliminate ⇨
• Thoracic duct: major lymph vessel, trunk in chest ⇨ veins (blood) ⇨ neck ⇨
• Heart (right) ⇨ blood cleansing organs

Outdoor exercise, fresh air strengthens immunity.
• Oxygen electrifies, kills bacteria, viruses

Dietary treatment: cold, flu
• CH. 6 (Lungs), CH. 20 (Cold, flu)

Case history #12. I (73): lacto-vegetarian, spices, exercise, etc. last 46 years: no colds, flus, flu shots, just occasional coughs, sore throats that cured quickly 1- 2 days via diet and herbs (licorice, cardamom, ginger).

The body is designed to be healthy. It will heal itself when given the opportunity (diet, rest, time, etc.). Most children in U.S. (1950's, 60's) contracted and cured **measles, chicken pox** (low death rate <1%) at home without doctors (no vaccines). No schools were shut down. Many parents believed these childhood diseases were necessary to strengthen immunity. Decades later, doctors and some parents decided these diseases were too dangerous that every child should be disease free, vaccinated, to protect all. If not, they were banned from most schools, despite being healthy. "No good deed (wisdom) goes unpunished." Too many vaccines can weaken immunity.

13. SKIN

Body's largest organ: solid, porous

1. Life-span: few weeks, renews

2. Holds, protects, helps regulate body temperature

3. External shield. Closed pores, retain heat protect against external entry: heat, cold, wind, viruses, etc. Open pores cool, vent heat, allow entry.

4. Two layers:

a) Epidermis (outer): nerve endings, dead cells, no blood vessels

b) Dermis (inner): several layers: blood, lymph vessels, hair follicles, nerves.

- Sudoriferous glands (millions): armpits, groin, except palms, soles of feet produce sweat/ perspiration (water, salt, urea) ⇨ pores (openings) ⇨ epidermis ⇨ cools the body

- Sebaceous glands: secrete sebum (oily liquid) ⇨ moistens, lubricates oils skin, hair; insulates, helps maintain body temperature, prevent sweat evaporation

5. Adipose tissue: connective tissue below skin, stores fat: insulation, energy reserve, produces histamine: anti-inflammatory

PATHOLOGIES:

A. Acne: inflammation of sebaceous glands: face, shoulders, back ⇨ raised, red skin eruptions, blackheads, pimples, pus

B. Hot, oily rashes (groin, armpits), shingles (CH. 25)

C. Boils: bacterial infection (sweat glands, hair follicles) ⇨ abscess, swelling, discharge (pus), pain, fever

D. Warts, moles, bumps under skin (face)

E. Psoriasis: skin, face, scalp, back, shoulders ⇨ dry, red, itchy, scaly, flaky skin. Case history: CH. 24

General causes:

1. Hormonal imbalances, drugs, cosmetics

2. Climate, bacteria, genetics

3. Diet: excess protein, fat, animal, fried foods, nut butters, chocolate, sugar ⇨
•   Thicken, heat, poison the blood ⇨ skin ⇨
•   Acne, rashes, boils, warts, psoriasis, etc.

Treatment: CMD #1, 2
•   Bitters: gotu kola (psoriasis), barberry (acne, boils), burdock, gentian
•   Coriander (rashes), turmeric, aloe: internal or topical: rashes, wounds, sores
•   Neem oil: acne, psoriasis, ringworm, jock itch
•   Avoid caffeine, sour foods, drinks
•   +/- M.D.

F. Eczema: thin, dry, cracked, red, inflamed skin ⇨ blisters ⇨ itch, weep, release fluid, form crust, scale, or flake

General dietary cause:
•   Deficient building, excess sugar (any)

Treatment: HMD (no red meat)
•   Cooked vegetables, spices (3- 7 per meal)
•   Neem oil, gotu kola, echinacea, golden seal

Case history #23. 1989, I (16 years' vegetarian, salads, fruit, sugar low protein, fat) ⇨ severe **eczema**: multiple blisters, cracked skin, bleeding, pus: all fingers ⇨ back of left hand ⇨ right. I read **Ayurvedic Healing** by Dr. Frawley, O.M.D., changed my diet (more protein, cooked vegetables, spices), cured, three weeks (CH. 21).

G. Acanthosis nigricans (AN): dry, itchy skin, dark velvety skin patches, tags via Diabetes (CH. 21)

H. Wrinkles

General causes:

1. Age, climate, cosmetics, sex

2. Diet: excess meat, salt, fermented foods, drinks

Treatment:
- Topical oils: olive, avocado, etc.
- Less salt, more fruit, vegetables

I. Cuts, burns, scarring

Treatment
- Astringents: self-heal, mullein or comfrey + little honey: stop bleeding
- Turmeric or calendula cream: burns, scarring

Case history #24. Knocked over a pot of boiling water onto my chest (+ tea shirt prolonged burning) ⇨ huge blister, **2nd degree burn**: diagnosed by paramedic. I washed it with salt water, applied calendula for several days ⇨ no scar.

J. Fungus: skin, toes, nails
- Neem, tea tree oil

K. Kidney yang deficiency (CH. 16)
- Bright white complexion

14. LOCOMOTION

Skeletal system
- Houses, protects, holds, moves the body

Anatomy, physiology
1. **Bones** (protein, fat, minerals), marrow (blood)
2. **Joints** two or more bones meet: stationary, mobile
3. **Cartilage** (gelatinous substance, shock absorber) caps, cushions, separates end of movable bones
4. **Ligaments** hold the bones are attached ⇔
5. **Tendons** (sinews) ⇔
6. **Muscles** (expand, contract)
7. Stimulated nourished via
8. **Nerves, jing** (CH. 16), **blood**, nutrients, etc.

Musculoskeletal diseases:
1. Rheumatoid Arthritis
2. Gout (uric acid)
3. Osteoarthritis: bone on bone, no cartilage
4. Restless Leg Syndrome, Plantar Fasciitis
5. Psoriatic Arthritis, Neuralgia, Sciatica
6. Phlebitis (clot: vein, leg)

General symptoms:
- Inflammation, pain, swelling, redness
- Stiffness, numbness, shaking

General causes:

1. Diet

a) Deficient protein, fat ⇨ extreme ⇨ thins, dries, weakens, inflames the bones, muscles, ligaments, etc. ⇨ #1, 4- 5

Treatment: HMD, turmeric

b) Excess protein, saturated fat, cholesterol ⇨ narrows arteries, decreases circulation, blood ⇨ arms, legs, bones, muscles, etc. ⇨ #2, 4- 6

c) Excess inorganic calcium (white flour, bread, cookies, chips, etc.), uric acid (CH. 22, Gout) ⇨ blood ⇨ joints: hips, knees, ankles ⇨ pain (migrates)

Treatment: CMD #1
- Apples, grapes, grapefruit, celery break down, eliminate uric acid, calcium deposits
- Pineapple: tendonitis
- Turmeric helps ligaments stretch, topical (cream): strained muscles, joints, sport injuries
- +/- M.D.

Case history #5. I (15- 54): bad knees via basketball and clogged arteries (excess building, animal) ⇨ limited movement, pain while walking, worse after game. In my 50's: water on the knees (swollen twice their size) 3x ⇨ drained (M.D.). Age 54, stopped playing, changed my diet: CMD #1, juices, one month to cure: no pain. Everything changes. Age 73, no pain.

Case history #25. I (69) excess white flour/ animal crackers ⇨ pain: up, down legs. I stopped, added celery (raw), grapes, grapefruit, cured.

2. Diuretics (water-pills), pharmaceutical. More info: case history #14 (CH. 19, Arthritis)

3. Injury, age

Osteoarthritis:
- No dietary cure
- Injectable gels (M.D.)

"A moving gate gathers no rust."

13. GLANDS

Organs (specialized cells) ⇨ produce hormones, digestive enzymes, wax, etc. generally not related to their own functions. Two types:

A. **Endocrine** (ductless): **hormones**: regulate functions of specific organs, groups of cells ⇨ pass directly into blood.

Two kinds:
- Steroids: estrogen, testosterone, cortisol
- Non-steroidal: anti-inflammatory

1. **Pineal** (unique: human beings): little known cone shaped organ in brain ⇨ melatonin: relaxant

2. **Pituitary** (brain): master gland, hormones:
- Growth, metabolism, stress, trauma
- Adrenal, thyroid, sex glands, hormones
- Skin pigmentation
- Autonomic nervous system regulates involuntary, vital functions: heart, circulation, etc.

a) Excess ⇨ gigantism, acromegaly: enlargement, elongation (hands, feet, face) in middle age

b) Deficiency ⇨ dwarfism (one cause)

3. **Thyroid** (base of neck, two lobes) ⇨ thyroxin ⇨ regulates metabolism (carbohydrates, protein, fat), growth, development, nervous system, body temperature

a) Deficient thyroxin, iodine ⇨ hypothyroidism ⇨
- Fatigue, cold intolerance, weight gain
- Muscle weakness, cramps; migraines
- Milky discharge (breast), painful menstruation
- Constipation, hair loss, scaly skin, insomnia
- Yellow orange discoloration: skin (palms, hands)

- Droopy, swollen eyes, yellow bumps (eyelids)
- Weak immunity, depression
- Mostly women: ages 30- 50

General causes:
- Deficient protein, fat, iodine
- Drugs, fluoride, pesticides, poisons, radiation
- Treatment: diet + M.D.

b) Deficient iodine ⇨ goiter: enlargement of thyroid (front of neck)
- Treatment: diet + M.D.

a) Excess iodine (kelp) ⇨ metallic taste, breath, decreases thyroxin

c) Thyroid disease (CH. 26)

4. **Thymus** (below thyroid): lymph, immune system. More info: CH. 10 (Immunity)

5. **Pancreas** ⇨ insulin, glucagon (regulate blood sugar), exocrine gland (CH. 7, Digestion)

6. **Adrenals** (sit atop kidneys)
- Cortex (outer part) ⇨ sex hormones, glucocorticoids, cortisone: carbohydrate, protein, fat metabolism; anti-inflammatory/ stress, essential to many bodily systems
- Medulla (inner most part) ⇨ mineral corticoids ⇨ maintain water and sodium balance.

7. **Sex glands**, gonads: ovaries, testes ⇨
- Reproductive hormones: Ch. 16

II. **Exocrine** (ducts ⇨ organs)
- Pancreas: digestive enzymes ⇨ SI
- Liver: bile ⇨ SI
- Skin, sweat, lacrimal (tears)
- Salivary, mammary, ears

16. REPRODUCTION

Reproduction is controlled by **jing**: sexual essence (ovum, sperm), **ojas** (Ayurveda, CH. 5): body's primary intelligent substance, fuel via parental pre-heaven, parental sexual essence (DNA, sperm, ovum) ⇨
- Combined with post-heaven essence (food) ⇨
- New jing (DNA, ovum, sperm) ⇨
- Governs birth, growth, reproduction ⇨

1. Stored in **left kidney** as kidney yin (material foundation, substance) ⇨

2. **Right kidney**: kidney yang (gate of fire) ⇨ motive force for all physiological processes ⇨ transforms kidney yin ⇨
- Marrow, brain, bones, spinal cord
- Adrenal, pituitary glands: sex hormones
- Ovaries ⇨ ovum, estrogen, progesterone
- Testes ⇨ sperm, testosterone
- Prostate: doughnut shaped, chestnut size male sex gland (encircles neck of urethra) ⇨ fluid, mixes with sperm ⇨ semen ⇨ sperm duct ⇨ urethra, penis

Kidney yin (substance) ⇨ root of heart, liver yin (CH. 5, TCM). Kidney yang (function, fire, transformation) ⇨ root of spleen, lung yang.

The amount of jing is limited, fixed at birth. You get one fuel tank. Jing ⇨

- **Fountain of youth**: strong bones, fertility, virility, immunity, rapid healing, lush colorful hair, deep sleep, moist, supple skin, etc. when full.

- Onset of **old age**: physical, mental decline, dryness, weakness, infertility, impotence, poor memory, balance, vision, etc. when low, in its decline: starts early: **men** (late teens), **women** (early 20's) but varies according to use.

The following decrease:

1. Old age
2. Heredity weakness via parents
3. Sex, orgasm daily, weekly (3x), worse when older or starting young
4. Masturbation: loss, no balance, exchange, mixing of opposing essences ⇨ weakness
5. Excessive or frequent childbirths

Sex: two edges sword: pleasurable, procreative but also weakness, death. Moderation or abstinence is recommended if not seeking procreation.

Recreational sex (men): withholding, forgoing orgasm via occasional contractions of anal sphincter muscles during sex ⇨ squeezes prostate, empties semen (testes) before it becomes full, swollen, stops urge to ejaculate ⇨ extends lovemaking, reduces loss of jing but can also strain, inflame when done incorrectly ⇨ extreme ⇨ cancer. A hot bath after soothes, relaxes prostate. Give up the small (daily, short orgasm, faster aging) for the greater (health, longevity, longer pleasure).

6. Chronic disease

7. Deficient protein, fat forces the body to consume jing as a replacement fuel decreases ovum, sperm, estrogen, testosterone, fertility.

Ayurveda (CH. 5): dairy, nuts, seeds, herbs (amla, ashwagandha) strengthen the reproductive organs. Meat, shellfish, eggs strengthen, but also excite, poison, irritate. Moderation. Avoid if kidneys are weak

Elephant tusks, rhinoceros' horns, tiger penis, shark fins, etc. **do not** increase jing, ojas, virility, longevity, much less justify **murder** of defenseless animals. Hunting for sport is murder.

Jing: never in excess ⇨ deficient with age use.

PATHOLOGIES

I. **Dietary**

A. **Long-term low protein**, **fat** ⇨ deficient, thin
blood, anemia ⇨ sex ⇨

1. Women ⇨
- Amenorrhea (CH. 19): delay, little or no period
- Decrease in estrogen
- PMS, dysmenorrhea, short-term pregnancy
- Frigidity: sexual passivity, inability to climax
- Miscarriage, infertility, early onset menopause
- Insufficient breast milk; dryness, fear

2. Men ⇨
- Low sperm, testosterone, premature ejaculation
- Impotence, sterility, spermatorrhea (leaking)

Blood (nutrients) via penile artery enlarges,
elevates, hardens the penis. **Testosterone** ⇨ nerves,
central nervous system ⇨ blood flow to penis ⇨ increases
sexual desire, ability to achieve, maintain an erection

Treatment: HMD
- Red meat, chicken, turkey, eggs, fish, garlic
- Dairy milk, ghee, butter, yogurt, sweet cheese
- Almonds, cashews, sesame seeds, chickpeas
- Mung, azuki beans, tofu, roots, sweet potatoes
- Dates, raisin, figs, bananas; spices (no peppers)
- Amla, ashwagandha, ginseng, licorice, lotus seed

1. Women:
- Evening primrose oil, nettle (estrogen)
- Saw palmetto berry (sweet, oily, astringent)
  strengthens digestion, absorption, helps cure
  small underdeveloped breasts, ovaries
- Siberian ginseng (digestion), royal jelly (jing)
- Breast milk (lack): saw palmetto berry, fennel,
  fenugreek seeds (gruel), nettles, grains
- Peppermint, parsley: stop lactation

- Breast feeding helps contract the uterus
- Avoid caffeine, tobacco, drugs ⇨ blood ⇨ breast milk ⇨ baby

2. Men:
- Saw palmetto: increases testosterone, potency; underdeveloped testicles, swollen prostate
- Ashwagandha, lotus seeds increase sperm

Both:
- Less, no sex (increases fertility, potency)
- +/- M.D.

B. **High protein**, **saturated fat**, **cholesterol**, animal, fried foods, hydrogenated oils, nut butters, etc. ⇨ blood ⇨ sex glands, organs

1. Women:
- PMS (CH. 24), dysmenorrhea
- Dark, red, purple blood, clots, pain
- Excessive menstrual flow: 7 days (+/-)
- Menorrhagia, metrorrhagia (CH. 23)
- Endometriosis (CH. 20)
- Tumors, cancer (breast, uterus): CH. 20

2. Men:
- Swollen, enlarged: benign prostatic hypertrophy
- Narrow arteries (legs, penis) ⇨ impotence (CH. 23), premature ejaculation, spermatorrhea
- Prostatitis: inflammation, pain, dysuria
- Tumors, cancer (CH. 24, Prostate)

Treatment: CMD #1, 2
- Spices: fennel, coriander, turmeric, saffron
- Bitters: aloe vera, gotu kola, dandelion
- Burdock: tumors: breasts, female sex organs
- Myrrh (uterus), ashwagandha (spermatorrhea)
- +/- M.D.

C. **Hormones** (natural, prescription, soy)

D. **Drugs**

E. **Kidney-Yin Deficiency**

General symptoms;
- Low grade afternoon fever, thirst
- Dry mouth, throat (night), night sweats
- Dizziness, tinnitus (low ringing), vertigo
- Deafness (kidneys open into ears)
- Sore back, nocturnal emissions
- Malar flush (partial facial flushing)
- Mental restlessness, insomnia
- Fear (cardinal sign), especially of falling
- Kidney yang deficiency

General causes:
- Chronic illness (liver, heart, lungs), overwork
- Excessive sexual activity especially during teenage years: depletes kidney essence
- Depletion of body fluids via febrile disease
- Overdose: Chinese herbal medicine (kidney yang)

Treatment: HMD or CMD #1
- Beef broth, duck, oyster, shellfish
- Milk, butter, cheese, chestnuts, sesame seeds
- Saw palmetto berry, ashwagandha, amla
- Women: Royal jelly, evening primrose oil, black currant oil, yarrow (estrogen, progesterone)
- Less or no sex
- +/- M.D.

VI. **Kidney-Yang Deficiency**

General symptoms (genito-urinary, chi deficiency):
- Aversion to cold, loose stools
- Weak, sore, lower back, knees, legs
- Abundant, frequent or scanty urination
- Weak-stream or dribbling after urination
- Incontinence, nocturia, spermatorrhea
- Edema (legs, ankles), bright white complexion

1. Women:
- PMS, dysmenorrhea, infertility
- Urinary tract, yeast infection (CH. 26)

- Leucorrhea: white vaginal discharge

2. Men
- Enlarged prostate (phlegm), impotence
- Premature ejaculation, spermatorrhea

General causes:

1. Chronic illness, old age, excessive sex, obesity

2. Cold, damp, low protein, fat diet, salads, fruit, juices, cold drinks, ice water, soda, smoothies

Treatment: CMD #2
- Beans, corn, carrots; parsley, black pepper
- Garlic, cloves, ginger, saffron: afternoon
- Myrrh (cleanses uterus) *

VII. **Kidney-Essence Deficiency**

1. Children: poor heredity constitution via parents (too old or poor health at conception) ⇨
- Poor bone development, late closure of fontanelle (baby's soft skull bones), mental dullness, retardation

2. Adults via old age, excessive sex ⇨
- Softening of bones, weak, sore back, legs, knees
- Sexual weakness, poor memory, loose teeth
- Premature loss or gray hair

Treatment (adults): HMD
- Ghee, kidneys, shrimp, coconut milk
- Chicken, turkey, meat, raspberry, cherries
- Almonds, cashews, sesame seeds, chickpeas
- Amla, ashwagandha, ginseng, licorice, lotus seed
- Saw palmetto berry, ashwagandha, no sex
- +/- M.D.

VIII. Miscellaneous

1. **Pregnancy**: HMD or CMD #1
- Vegetables: cooked > raw
- Avoid bitters (laxatives, diuretics, coffee), hot spices (peppers, garlic) ⇨ miscarriage
- Coffee, smoking ⇨ blood ⇨ fetus, breast milk

2. **Post-partum**: weakness, depression

Treatment: correct diet
- Vegetables (cooked > raw)
- Circulation, cleansing (uterus): myrrh, saffron, pennyroyal; avoid coffee, laxatives, diuretics
- Love, support +/- counseling

3. **Menopause**: 12 years after end of menstruation (45- 55) ⇨ dual decline: jing, blood ⇨
- Fatigue, depression, bloating, headaches
- Insomnia, dry skin, vagina, hot flashes (CH. 22)
- Muscle, joint pain, osteoporosis, hysteria
- Duration varies (1- 10 years): health, diet, etc.

Anemia, excess sex, caffeine, smoking; deficient protein, fat accelerates onset and severity of symptoms.

General treatment:
- Diet via constitution (Ayurveda, CH. 5):
- Vata (air): old age, depression, anxiety, insomnia
- Pitta (fire): frequent hot flashes, anger, irritability
- Kapha (water): edema, weight gain, sleepiness
-
- Hot flashes: pear juice + peppermint tea; progesterone cream, yarrow
- Myrrh, aloe gel (P, K), ashwagandha
- Hysteria: gotu kola, valerian, chamomile

4. **Hysterectomy**

Uterus (organ) controls, houses reproduction, emotions, and creativity (Ayurveda). Removal ⇨
- Emotional imbalance, feelings of insecurity
- Depression, anxiety, anger, fear
- Lower metabolism, weight gain

Treatment: middle diet adjusted accordingly
- After surgery: turmeric, Arjuna (Ayurveda)
- Tonic herbs: aloe vera, saffron, dang gui
- Calming, nervine herbs: gotu kola, valerian

5. **Anal sex**
1. Feces, poisons (LI) ⇨ penis ⇨ kidneys ⇨ bacterial infections ⇨ blood ⇨ monkey pox, AIDS, etc.
2. Weakens, loosens the anus, sphincter muscles ⇨ leaks jing, ojas (CH. 5, 16) ⇨ aging, weak immunity.

17. DISEASE, DIAGNOSIS & TREATMENT

There are many ways to diagnose and treat disease.

Just as an auto mechanic, diagnoses and treats a car, according to its parts, so does a doctor/ physician diagnose and treat the body mind via its parts, each of which performs functions in association with other parts.
- Nerves, nervous system ⇨ electrical impulses
- 7 glands, 10 organs, hormones, blood, acid, enzymes, mucus, antibodies ⇨ digestion, respiration, circulation, elimination, locomotion immunity, reproduction, vision, memory, etc.

Naturopathic medicine (East, West) diagnoses and treats disease via nutritional, energetic/material analysis, as every diseased structure has an overall hot, cold, thick, thin, solid, hollow, watery, etc. nature construction, operation caused in general by poor diet:
- Too much or too little **building** (protein, sat. fat, cholesterol, EFA, animal, plant, **cleansing** (fruit, vegetables, juices, water)
- Excess fat, flour, sugar, raw, etc.

Each disease, tissue, vessel, hormone, blood, stone, tumor, cancer, virus has a specific poor diet, nutrient, energetic, material nature that can be stopped and replaced with more of the opposite nutritional, energetic, etc. nature is the essence of naturopathic treatment.

Western, allopathic medicine (drugs, surgery, radiation) uses blood, hormone analysis (nutrients, hormones, etc.), x-rays, etc. to diagnose disease.

Body (health, disease): generally easy to diagnose and control via diet, herbs, exercise, sun, earth due to its size and material nature, **composition** (elements, nutrients, poisons), **construction** (thick, thin, dry, watery, solid, hollow, etc.) ⇨ ongoing predictable and mostly controllable product of **cause and effect**, balance of opposites via **changes** in energy ⇨

1. Sun, earth, water, plants, oxygen, carbon dioxide
2. Animal, plant food (building, cleansing nutrients)
3. Herbs, coffee, alcohol, drugs, preservatives
4. Pollution, exercise, sex, smoking, age, etc.
- Create, build, fuel, heat, cool, dry, air, moisten
- Increase, decrease, purify, preserve or destroy
- Daily, slowly, quickly, small to large ⇨

30 trillion cells (30,000 billion) ⇨ billions (1,000 million) ⇨ **tissues**: nerves (3 trillion), glands, organs, bones, muscles, skin; arteries, veins, capillaries (10 billion); hormones, blood, acid, enzymes, antibodies, mucus, urine, stool **functions** physical, mental **healthy**, **diseased**, stone, tumor, cancer, etc.

Most bodily disease has **multiple** causes (#1- 3) and effects (symptoms), some that can be changed, eliminated; others not. **Poor diet** (too much, too little building, cleansing, overeating, undereating, late meals, processed foods, etc.) tends to dominate. Most diet-related if not too severe can be cured via **correct diet**, herbs which is why myself and others were able to **cure**:
- Atherosclerosis, high blood pressure, angina, eczema
- Arthritis, Restless Leg Syndrome, Plantar Fasciitis
- Common cold, sore throat, sour body odor, insomnia
- Obesity, poor vision, impotence, sore lower back
- GIRD, Irritable Bowel Syndrome, anal fissure, anxiety
- Psoriasis, edema, cellulite, sinusitis, neuralgia, ADD
- Anemia, miscarriage, UTI, yeast infection, Crohn's
- Diabetes mellitus (adult onset), tumors, cancer (breast)

All diets, dietary diseases are defined by individual and collective foods, nutrients: building cleansing.

1. **Building** nutrients: protein (water-soluble), saturated fat, cholesterol, EFA: animal, plant
2. **Cleansing** nutrients: water, minerals, vitamins; sugar, starch/ fiber: fruit, vegetables

Correct balance, kinds, amounts ⇨ **health**. Incorrect, greater (>) or lesser (<) amounts, kinds ⇨ **extreme** (varies: condition, climate) ⇨ **disease** (one cause)

Excess protein, saturated fat, cholesterol, protein ⇨
- Blood clots, high cholesterol, plaque, narrow, clogged arteries, high blood pressure, heart disease, insomnia, Peripheral Artery Disease (PAD), arthritis, Plantar Fasciitis, Restless Leg
- Obesity, psoriasis, ADD, impotence
- PMS, dysmenorrhea, stones, tumors, cancer

Deficient protein, fat (animal, plant) ⇨
- Arthritis, Restless Leg, Plantar Fasciitis, PAD
- Insomnia, neuralgia, anemia, ADD, impotence
- PMS, dysmenorrhea, infertility, miscarriage
- Thin, dry, cracked skin, eczema, fatigue

Ayurveda: **three** dietary, nutritional, energetic disease extremes:

1. **Pitta**, excess building, fire, protein, saturated fat, cholesterol, animal, spicy, sour, salty, fried foods ⇨ thick, hard, hot, dry, watery, infection

2. **Vata**, deficient building, excess cleansing, air ⇨ thin, dry, cold, weak, shaky, inflamed

3. **Kapha**, excess water, sugar, fat, fruit, juices, sodas, cold drinks, dairy, mucus, phlegm

Every disease grows or deteriorates via favorite (life) and non-favorite (death) nutrients, foods, herbs, etc.

Treatment plan (days, months, etc.)
1. Reduce or eliminate the offending extreme, favorite disease foods, nutrients, herbs, etc.
2. Do more of the opposite foods, herbs, etc. until health is restored.

Correct diet varies according to dietary cause, severity of condition and climate. Some diseases have singular dietary causes, others, multiple. The same diet, foods that help reverse, eliminate, **cure** one disease, variation may **worsen**, grow another.

A. Musculoskeletal diseases ⇨ inflammation, pain, swelling, stiffness, numbness, deterioration shaking, ⇨ bones, ligaments, muscles, nerves ⇨
1. Rheumatoid arthritis
2. Gout (uric acid)
3. Osteoarthritis (bone on bone)
4. Restless Leg Syndrome, Neuralgia
5. Plantar Fasciitis (PF), Sciatica
6. Psoriatic arthritis

General causes:

1. Diet (nutrients) build, fuel, moisten, cleanse, etc.

a) Deficient protein, fat ⇨ extreme ⇨ weakens, dries nerves, bones, ligaments, muscles ⇨ #1, 4- 5
• Treatment: HMD, turmeric

b) Excess protein, saturated fat, cholesterol ⇨ thick, narrow, clogged arteries, veins ⇨ decreased circulation, blood ⇨ legs ⇨ dries, tightens, weakens, pains, etc. ⇨ #2, 4- 6
• Treatment: CMD #1

c) Excess processed, "enriched" white flour: inorganic calcium ⇨ blood ⇨ joints, muscles, etc. ⇨ pain (fixed, migrating)
• Treatment: grapes, celery, eliminate white flour

Musculoskeletal symptoms via anemia, clogged arteries: sometimes misdiagnosed, treated as Multiple Sclerosis: Pharmaceutical Drugs (CH. 24)

2. Injury, drugs, age, sports

B. PMS, dysmenorrhea, impotence, insomnia via
• Excess or deficient protein, fat

Climate
1. Cold climates generally require more building, animal, cooking and less cold, raw, juices.

2. Hot: generally, less animal, more cleansing

Many diseases are difficult to diagnose, especially if confusing, opposing symptoms or ignorance of anatomy.

Case history #8. Woman (60, vegetarian, FL), **anxiety** (CH. 19), occasional yelling during consultation, seemed to be overheated despite "cold" diet, salads, low protein, fat, fuel. She was deficient, weak, not enough protein, fat to control, moisten, cool her normal energy, fire, emotions which would occasionally rage out of control. I recommended the HMD, which was a problem (vegetarian). She compromised (veal, eggs). Three days later, she called, very happy, all anxiety attacks gone, having great bowel movements, etc.

Obesity or excess waste in LI ⇨ pushes down on urinary bladder (UB) ⇨ urgency to urinate ⇨ misdiagnosed, treated (drugs, surgery): prostate, kidney, UB disease (CH. 24, Pharmaceutical Drugs).

Curing times vary:

1. **Acute, rapid onset** (common cold, sprain): generally curable, day 1, 2 depending on health.

2. **Chronic** disease takes time, months, years to develop and consequently time to cure, if curable.

Three dietary diseases, treatment plans
- +/- M.D.

A. Excess Building: protein, saturated fat, cholesterol: red meat, chicken, turkey, fried foods, ice cream, butter, hydrogenated oils, etc. ⇨
- Clots, plaque, atherosclerosis, arteriosclerosis
- High blood pressure, red face, angina, insomnia
- Arthritis, gout, liver, gall bladder disease
- Tumors, cancer, stones, acne, rashes, psoriasis
- UTI, PMS, dysmenorrhea, prostatitis, impotence

Treatment: CMD #1, 2

B. Deficient building, protein, fat (animal, plant) ⇨
•   Anemia, amenorrhea, PMS, dysmenorrhea
•   Infertility, miscarriage, impotence, low libido
•   Low blood pressure, autoimmune, emaciation
•   Colds, flu, shaking, numbness, arthritis, neuralgia
•   Dizziness, forgetfulness, premature aging, fear
•   Children (deficient EFA): poor mental development

Treatment: HMD, animal, nuts, seeds, etc.

C. Excess water, sugar, dairy, fruit, juice, smoothies,
    cold drinks, ice water, sodas, etc. ⇨
•   Gas, bloating, excessive urination, loose stools
•   Mucus (lungs) ⇨ coughing, shortness of breath,
    sinusitis, bronchitis, sleep apnea, cold, flu
•   Stones, UTI, leucorrhea, yeast infection, Candida

Treatment: CMD #2
•   Cooked vegetables, bitter, astringent herbs

SIMPLE ENERGETIC DIAGNOSIS:
1. Fold a piece of paper in half
2. List, separate diet, herbs, etc. ⇨

Hot, building	Cold, cleansing
Red meat, pork, fish	Water
Chicken, turkey	Vegetables, fruit
Nuts, seeds, beans	Juices (+ pulp)
Fried, fermented, sour	Smoothies, sodas
Raw onions, chili	Sugar (all)
Cooked, boiled, baked	Soda, smoothies
Herbs: spices, sour	Bitter, sweet, astringent
Salt, alcohol, coffee	Minerals
Hot climate	Cold climate

Examine the list and identify the imbalance. One side will always be greater. This is your energetic profile. If you feel, look and act well, then your diet, balance is correct, healthy. If not, you need to change, do more of the opposite until well.

This is a simple diagnosis, treatment plan that may work if the disease is not too complicated. Complicated, confusing symptoms require greater knowledge (biology) as every structure, function healthy, diseased has specific favorite (growth, life) and non-favorite (dissolution, death) foods, raw, cooked, nutrients, herbs, climates, etc.

General diagnosis, symptoms:

I. Chi, blood, body fluids, jing, wind

A. Chi (Qi): four major pathologies (CH. 4)

1. **Chi deficiency**
- Fatigue, shallow breathing, weak voice
- Feels cold, catches cold, sweats easily
- Palpitations, pale tongue, no appetite
- Chi stagnation, rebellion

2. **Chi Stagnation**
- Depression, mood swings, dark, purple tongue
- Frequent sighing, gloomy feeling, irritability
- Distention: chest, abdomen, muscle pain

3. **Chi Rebellion**
- Burping, nausea, vomiting, hiccoughs
- Heartburn, headaches, restlessness

4. **Sinking chi**
- Heaviness, downward bearing sensation
- Varicose veins, depression, prolapse
- Incontinence, spermatorrhea (leaking sperm)

B. Blood

1. **Deficient, thin** (low protein, fat)
- Pale face, tongue, lips, fatigue, insomnia
- Pain, inflammation, numbness, shaking
- Dry lips, eyes, skin; dizziness, forgetfulness
- Amenorrhea, infertility, miscarriage, impotence

2. **Stagnation**
- Dark complexion, purple lips, nails
- Clots, atherosclerosis, high blood pressure
- Tumors, cancer, obesity, poor circulation
- Inflammation, arthritis, fixed, stabbing pain
- Swollen organs, PMS, dysmenorrhea

3. **Heat**
- Bleeding, easily bruises, insomnia
- Toxic blood: acne, boils, psoriasis, itching

C. Body fluids (mucus, sweat, etc.)

1. **Deficiency**
- Dry skin, muscles, mouth, throat, eyes, etc.
- Dry stools, scanty urination

2. **Excess**
- Mucus, phlegm, snoring, sleep apnea
- Edema, cellulite, sweet body odor
- Loose stools, excessive urination
- Phlegm nodules: thyroid, lymph gland

D. Jing: **deficiency** (only in decline)
- Premature aging, graying, loss of hair
- Bone loss (osteoporosis), night sweats
- Impotence, infertility, dementia

E. Wind (air) ⇨
- Stiffness, numbness, spasms, tremors
- Vertigo, dizziness, loss of balance, pain
- Parkinson's Disease

II. Organs

Lungs
- Mucus, phlegm, cough, shortness of breath
- Asthma, sleep apnea, cold, flu, bronchitis
- Oxygen deprivation, fatigue, depression
- Immunity

Heart
- Palpitations, tachycardia, cold limbs
- Chest, left arm pain, insomnia
- Red face, red bulbous nose

Spleen
- Indigestion, loose stools, indecision, worry

Stomach
- Nausea, vomiting, reflux, halitosis
- Dry tongue, mouth, burning lips
- GIRD, heartburn, ulcer, frontal headache

Small Intestine
- Abdominal pain, bloating, nausea
- Malabsorption, acidity, insomnia

Pancreas
- Hypoglycemia, hyperglycemia, diabetes
- Dry mouth, irritability, insomnia, neuralgia
- Fatigue, headache, dizziness, sweating, nausea
- Nausea, palpitations, tremors, anxiety, confusion
- Swollen feet, constant hunger, blurred vision

Liver
- Inability to digest fat, tinnitus (loud)
- Red eyes, blurred vision, floaters
- Temporal headache, shoulder, neck tension
- Pain in abdomen: right flank, bloated
- Anger, irritability, loud voice, insomnia

Gall bladder
- Nausea, vomiting fluids, bitter taste
- Stones, jaundice, piercing pain: right side

Kidneys
- Weak, sore lower back, knees, edema (ankles)
- Dysuria, incontinence, stones, insomnia, fear
- Dry mouth, throat at night, night sweats
- Cold body, limbs; pale, white complexion

Urinary Bladder
- Stones, painful, burning urination, UTI

Large intestine
- Malabsorption, loose stools
- Constipation, hemorrhoids, diverticulitis

Tongue diagnosis: stomach fluids overflow onto tongue ⇨ thin, white, moist coating.
1. Excess cold foods, drinks ⇨ thick white, moist coating
2. Fluid, blood, jing deficiency ⇨ red, thin, dry, no coating +/- shaking
3. Excess building ⇨ thick, yellow coating
4. Late meals, snacks ⇨ dry mouth, tongue

Gender, age (general tendencies)

1. Women: watery, cold, deficient (menstruation) generally need more building, protein, fat, cooked vegetables, spices but can become dry, thin via too little protein, fat.

2. Men: hot, fiery (testosterone) generally need more fruit, vegetables, less building, animal, spices, alcohol, coffee but can become weak via too little protein, fat or damp via kapha diet.

3. Elderly (vata): dry, weak, airy generally require dairy, cooked vegetables +/ eggs, chicken.

There are many ways to diagnose. I recommend:

1. **Dictionary of Medical Terms** Mikel A. Rothenberg, M.D. & Charles F. Chapman Barron's Educational Series, Inc., paperback (7" x 4")

2. **Prescription for Nutritional Healing** Phyllis Balch, CNC, James F. Balch, M.D.

3. **Internet**

4. **M.D.**, blood tests, x rays, etc. are an accurate diagnosis, sees what the naked eye cannot.

Allopathic doctors (M.D.), drugs, surgery, radiation while important, and many times life-saving ⇨

a) May cure, eliminate the effect (disease, symptoms), but generally not cure, remove cause, which is why history, most disease repeats itself in one form, location or another.

b) Do not know or openly admit the cause of most disease (most textbooks: cause unknown), yet more than willing to try drugs, surgery, etc. Has your doctor ever said, diet causes most disease?

c) Always advertise (last 100+ years): real "cure," new drug, etc. is "**just around the corner**."

d) Use fear to demean, discourage patient responsibility, independence. "If you do not take the COVID vaccine, you may suffer serious complications, die or worse, infect, kill your grandparents, children, etc."

e) Harmful (CH. 23, Iatrogenic Disease)

f) Not the only medicine, first treatment

Total reliance or avoidance of allopathy, naturopathy, nutritionists, dieticians, herbalists, etc. can also be dangerous, as every medicine has its positives and negatives.

Self-education, books, dietary changes, health, sickness is your best, most vivid control.

18. COOKING CLASS

Healthy food should always taste good. Welcome to the world's shortest cooking class, based on the middle diet meal plan, 3 variations and herbs (CH. 1, 3, 16).

1. **Colder middle diet #1**
- Lacto-vegetarian, vegetables (raw > cooked), fruit
- Tastes, herbs: sweet, bitter, astringent
- Reduce, eliminate excess building, fire

2. **Colder middle diet #2**
- Vegan, beans, grains, vegetables (cooked), etc.
- Tastes, herbs: pungent (spices), bitter, astringent
- Reduce, eliminate excess fluids, mucus, fat

3. **Hotter middle diet**
- Animal, nuts, seeds, grains, vegetables (cooked, roots, ground), oil, salt; fermented foods, fruit
- Tastes, herbs: sweet, sour, salty, spices
- Tonify, eliminate deficiency, dryness, coldness

The best, healthiest cook, restaurant in general is you in your own kitchen, controlling all the ingredients (organic, fresh, etc.), mood, atmosphere, etc. If you can buy, wash, cut vegetables, boil water, add spices, grind nuts, seeds, follow a recipe, keep track of time and taste what you eat, then you are ready, qualified. You will need a minimum of 10- 60 minutes per meal.

Variety is important, however most vegetables, fruits, grains, nuts, seeds, etc. have similar a similar nutrients make-up. The following are nutrient rich:
1. Apples, oranges, dates, raisins, pineapple
2. Beets, carrots, squash, yams, potatoes, onions
3. Lettuce, celery, broccoli, cabbage, cauliflower
4. Rice, barley, oats, millet, noodles, bread
5. Azuki, mung beans, lentils, chickpeas, tofu
6. Walnuts, almonds, sesame, pumpkin seeds

Best quality food, herbs, vitality, nutrition, aroma, taste: **organically grown** via environmentally, earth friendly fertilizers: grass, produce, manure and no artificial fertilizers, pesticides, preservatives, dyes, etc.
- 20%+ more expensive. Less expensive:
a) Sale or bulk (3- 5#). Carrots, potatoes, onions, fruit, etc., refrigerated: longer lasting
b) Online: walnuts: $12/lb., grocery stores $20

Most corporate, large farms: high artificial chemicals. Smaller farms: less. Washing removes some external water-soluble poisons (skin), but not internal.

Free range, grain, grass fed animals (no antibiotics, preservatives, etc.): healthier, tastier, more nutritious > commercial

Freshly prepared food: greater nutrition, vitality, aroma, taste > day old, frozen, canned, dried, highly processed, preserved, salted

Running, filtered **water** (less fluoride, chlorine, toxins, etc.): best quality, vitality, nutrition, taste; bottled water, less. Plastic bottles may leak microplastics. Only 15% of all plastic is recycled There are many good filters available. Avoid distilled water (leaches minerals), exception: kidney stones.

The best diet can become the worst, as **all food, nutrients not digested, absorbed become poisons, waste.** For maximize digestion, nutrient absorption:

1. **Smaller** meals. Stomach: ½ solid food, ¼ liquid, ¼ space to fully digest, mix acid, enzymes.
- Overeating: per or between meals decreases digestion, absorption, increases weight.

2. **Order** of eating, taste per meal
- Beginning: fruit, desserts (+/-), sweet
- Middle: protein, fat, vegetables, salt, spices, sour
- End: +/- salad +/- tea (bitter, astringent)

3. Eat more: **day** (digestion stronger, body upright, active than **night** (less active, sitting, lying down) ⇨ slows, stagnates movement of food

4. **Spices** in varying degrees stimulate the stomach, pancreas, small intestine, liver ⇨ acid, enzymes, bile ⇨ improve digestion, nutrient absorption, circulation, immunity, decrease mucus

5. More info: CH. 7 (Digestion)

Cooking   classes (informative,   social)   and cookbooks are essential: taste, nutrition

General cooking times, proportions:

1. Meat: fresh: 30 min. +/- size, frozen (longer), eggs (7 min. +/-)

2. Beans: 30- 60 min. (soaking overnight decreases cooking time) generally 2 parts water: 1 bean. Bean squish easily when properly cooked

3. Whole grains (25– 60 min.): 2 water: 1 grain; cracked (5 min.), noodles (5- 10) less water

• Water proportions, cooking times vary: stove (gas, electric, etc.), cookware

4. Nuts, seeds: raw ground (nut, seed mill, coffee grinder), 3 TB/ meal, if no other protein.

5. Vegetables: 3/ meal
a) Roots: potatoes, carrots, beets (7- 10 min.)
b) Ground: broccoli, celery, cauliflower, cabbage, onion (5)
c) Leaves: kale, collard greens, watercress (2- 5)
• Smaller cuts (matchsticks, slivers, diced) cook faster; larger: slower
• Cook at same time: layer: onions on bottom (more heat, cooks faster) > roots ⇨ ground ⇨ leaves

6. Condiments

a) Salt (NaCl): sea, rock: best quality, high trace
   minerals. Sodium (Na): minimum daily
   requirement: 1,500- 2,300 mg.
- 1 tsp. salt (2,300), medium stalk, celery (32),
- 1 oz. Swiss cheese (54), 6 oz. sirloin steak (96)

b) Bragg's Liquid Aminos (non-alcohol soy sauce, 1
   tsp. = 310 mg sodium)

Avoid excess salt, spices ⇨ indigestion, overeating,
thirst, drinking. Dominant taste in every meal: sweet
(healthiest). Adding ground nuts, seeds or peanut butter
to broth (cooked vegetables, especially sweet, carrots,
parsnips, sweet potatoes, yams, onions, etc.) at end of
cooking, heat, burner turned off ⇨ increases sweet taste
⇨ decreases desire for excess salt and hot spices:

Cookware: cast iron, stainless steel, enamelware,
glass pots, wooden cooking utensils (less noisy). Avoid
Teflon, aluminum ⇨ scratch, chip easily, spread
hazardous chemicals into food. Pots with thicker bottoms
evenly distribute the heat. Thin: easily burn, cook faster.

Serving sizes (individual), water proportions, cooking
times, stoves (gas, electric, etc.) vary. **All cooking**: (1)
bring to boil, (2) cover, lower flame: simmer (light boil).

I. Breakfast menus (C= cup)

A. **Fruit or juice**: pitta, excess building

B. **Oatmeal, carrots, walnuts**: pitta, vata (3 min.)
1. Add ¼ C oat flakes (rolled), ¼ tsp. sea salt to ¾
   C water. Cover, simmer 3 minutes.
2. Add ¼ C grated raw, organic carrots; ground
   walnuts (2 TB), raisins (1 TB), cinnamon, black
   pepper, Braggs Aminos or tabasco sauce. Serve.
- Raw carrots, beets (sweet) reduce spicy taste
- Do not eat more than 3x/ week: purines (gout)

Soft cereals, grains (greater, 2- 3x water, cooking time): easier to digest.

C. **Vegetable omelet**: vata, deficiency (12 min.)
1. Sautee: ¼ C each: broccoli, carrot, celery, onion (sliced thin) in 1 TB vegetable oil, 5 min.
2. Add, scramble 2 eggs; cook 7 min. +/-
3. Add black pepper, coriander, turmeric
4. Serve, finish with herb tea or coffee.

D. Precooked **chicken** or **turkey, vegetables** (raw, cooked): vata, blood deficiency (15 minutes)
1. ¼ C: sweet potato, 1 C water. Simmer 10 min.
2. Add broccoli, celery, cook 3- 5 min.
3. Mix with chicken (turkey), chopped romaine lettuce, black pepper, coriander. Serve.

E. **Corn, potatoes, carrots, celery**: P, K (10)
1. ¼ C each: corn (fresh, frozen), potatoes (white, sweet), carrot in 1 C water. Cook 7 min.
2. Add ¼ C raw celery or romaine lettuce: crunchy
3. Add 1 TB peanut butter (dilute in broth), black pepper +/- 1 tsp. each: Bragg's. Serve.

II. Soups (vegan)

A. **Tofu vegetable**: pitta, vata (7 min.)
1. Add ¼ C each: tofu, carrot, broccoli to 1 C water. Cook 5 min.
2. Add ¼ C celery. Cook 1 min.
3. Add 2 TB sunflower seeds or walnuts (extra protein, crunch) + cumin, coriander, fennel. Braggs. Garnish with parsley. Serve

B. **Lentil, corn, vegetable**: P, V, K (30 min.)
1. Add ¼ C lentils, 1 C water. Simmer 23 min.
2. Add onions, corn (frozen), potato (thin cut), ¼ tsp. salt. Cook 5 min. Add celery. Cook 2 min.
3. Mix with ground walnuts; spices (black pepper, coriander, cumin, etc.), Braggs or miso (1 tsp.).
4. Garnish with parsley. Serve.

C. **Noodles, vegetables**: pitta (10)
- Noodles (instructions) + lettuce, cooked celery, broccoli, peanut butter (1 TB), black pepper

III. Lunch, dinner menus (mostly vegetarian)

A. **Brown rice**, **walnuts**, vegetables: V, P, K (45+)

Cooking pot #1
1. ¼ C brown rice, ¾- 1 C water, ¼ tsp. salt. Simmer 45 minutes +/-.
- Variation: millet or pearl barley (¼ C): 1 C water, ¼ tsp. salt. Simmer 30 minutes +/-.

Cooking pot #2
1. Add ¼ C each: carrot (sliced), corn, 1½ C water. Cook 8 min. Add ¼ C celery. Cook 2 min.
2. Add chopped lettuce, ground walnuts (or pecans) or seeds; cumin, fennel, coriander, Braggs
3. Mix with pot #1.

B. **Adzuki beans**, **barley**, vegetables: P, K (60)

Cooking pot #1
1. Add ¼ C each: adzuki beans, barley (soak both overnight) to 2 C of water. Cover, simmer 55 min. until beans soft (easily squish between fingers). Add ¼ tsp. salt. Simmer 2- 3 min.

Cooking pot #2
1. Add ¼ C each: broccoli, carrot, cauliflower to 1½ C water. Simmer 3- 5 min.
2. Add ¼ C lettuce, pinches: cumin, turmeric, coriander, Braggs. Mix with pot #1.

C. **Millet, tempeh stew**: kapha (25 min.)

Cooking pot #1
1. Add ¼ C of millet, ¼ tsp. salt: 1 C water.
2. Cover, simmer 25 min.

Cooking pot #2
1. Tempeh (3 ounces), 3 mushrooms (presoak ½ hour), 1½ C water. Cook 10 min.
2. Add ¼ C each: broccoli, cauliflower. Cook 3 min.
3. Add celery (¼ C diced), ground sunflower seeds, cumin, coriander, black pepper, Braggs.
4. Mix with pot #1. Serve.

D. **Basmati rice, mung beans**, vegies: P/ K (27)

Cooking pot #1
1. ¼ C white basmati rice, mung beans, 1½ C water simmer 25 min. Add ¼ tsp salt. Cook 2 min.

Cooking pot #2
1. ½ C each: broccoli, celery, cauliflower, 1 C water. Simmer 3- 5 min.
2. Add spices, Braggs, walnuts
3. Mix with pot #1

E. **Polenta** (cooked corn meal), tofu, walnuts, vegetables: P, K (8 min.). One pot.
1. ½" polenta, ½ C each: potato, onion (cubed), 1 C water. Simmer 8 min.
2. Mix with ¼ C raw celery, salad greens, 2 TB walnuts, ¼ tsp. black pepper, Braggs. Serve.

F. **Swiss cheese** (or pre-cooked chicken, turkey, red meat) + vegetables: vata (6 min.). One pot.
1. ¼ C each: green bean, bell pepper (sliced), ½ C water. Simmer 6 min.
2. Add Swiss cheese, celery, romaine lettuce; cardamom, coriander, cumin +/- mustard. Serve.

G. **Salad**: spinach, celery, lettuce, carrots, etc. +/- dressing (diluted, 1 TB peanut butter, etc.): Pitta
• **Sandwich**: one slice of bread (whole wheat, rye) cut in half. Add mustard. It fills the stomach, which decreases hunger as well as craving for sweets.

H. **Vegetable meal:** raw, grated beets, carrots, lettuce, celery, mix with well-cooked onions, lightly cooked cauliflower. At end, dissolve 1 TB peanut butter in broth of cooked vegetables +/- nuts, spices, hot sauce, Braggs.

I. **Restaurants** (occasional): American, Asian, Chinese, etc. that serve vegetables (variety). Enjoy, break the monotony. Avoid salad bars (contamination: hands, coughing).

IV. Desserts (not a feature of every meal)

a) **Cookies**: add precooked: baked yam (without skin), pumpkin, hard squash or raw grated carrot + ginger, cinnamon to organic cookie mix. Bake. Sweet vegetables replace sugar. My good friend Marcia came up with the idea.

b) **Toast**, **jelly** (sugar free)

c) **Bread** (1 slice), 1 TB each **peanut butter**, **raisins**, ¼ tsp: cinnamon, ginger, fold in half: healthier, fresher than packaged cookies.

d) **Cous cous cake** (serves 2): ½ C each: cous cous, apple juice + 2 TB each: raisins, walnuts, ½ tsp cinnamon. Bring to a boil; turn off, cover and refrigerate 15 minutes to form.

e) Cook 1 **apple** (cored), cut in pieces, 2 TB **raisins**, cinnamon in ¼ C water, light boil: 2 minutes

f) Ice cream substitute: **yogurt** (low fat, plain, unsweetened) + honey or maple syrup + cardamom, cinnamon.

g) **Snacks**: raisins, raw carrot, celery, lettuce. You make the rules, habits.

h) Junk food. Sometimes a little junk food (candy, cookies, etc.) is necessary. Buy small amounts. The healthier you eat, feel, the lesser tolerance, desire, taste for junk. Filling the stomach with fruit, vegetables, yogurt reduces appetite and sugar craving.

V. Herb tea (CH. 3) after meal increases digestion

1. **Peppermint** (mild spicy). Sit 1 minute in boiled water, then remove tea bag.

2. **Hawthorn berry** (sour), increases digestion, lowers cholesterol, blood pressure.

3. **Green** (sour, bitter), slight trace of caffeine digests fat, lowers cholesterol. All bitters on empty stomach cause nausea. Do not flavor with sugar, sweeteners (reduces fat cleansing).

4. **Chamomile** (bitter, pungent) digests fat, good for children.

The kitchen is your best friend, digestive system, transforms food into blood. Keep it clean. Always have a good attitude, gratitude and peace when cooking, eating, as bad attitude, emotions, disruptive, loud music ⇨ indigestion.

Section II. Diseases A- Z

This section focuses primarily on dietary cause +/- sex, climate, age, etc.

Dietary, herbal therapy takes **time** (days, months) as it slowly builds and cleanses. Organic foods: fastest healing. The older, less active you get, the faster bad habits, foods cause disease, the slower the cure.

Herbs (CH. 3): use some not all. Less is more.
1. Short-term use: daily, 2x/day, 1- 3 weeks +/-
2. Long-term (spices, tonic, sweet herbs, longer)
3. Manufacturer's directions, internet, etc.
4. Discontinue when heathy
5. Organic: best quality when available
6. Generally powerless without corresponding dietary changes.
7. May conflict with prescription drugs. Consult M.D.

Best books, education:
1. **Yoga of Herbs** Dr. David Frawley, O.M.D., Dr. Vasant Lad
2. **The Energetics of Western Herbs, Volumes I, II** Peter Holmes

19. "A" DISEASES

Acne

Inflammatory disease of skin, sebaceous glands (secrete sebum, oil) ⇨ face, shoulders, back ⇨
- Red, raised skin, bumps, nodules, cysts, scarring
- Blackheads, hard, painful, oily pimples, pus

General causes:

1. Age, hormones, cosmetics

2. Diet: high dairy, sugar, saturated fat, trans fats/ hydrogenated oils) increase inflammation, oil stimulating hormones.

Treatment: CMD #2
- Barberry, burdock, gentian; neem oil (topical)
- More info: CH. 13 (Skin)

Addiction

Addiction is a choice ⇨ seeking happiness via drugs, alcohol ⇨ strong or irresistible dependence ⇨ physical, mental "high," but also eventual pain, disease, destructive behavior, etc. Everyone seeks happiness in one form or another. Some happiness is short, quick, turns into opposite, poison, pain, others, longer lasting.

Allopathic medicine (M.D.) prescribes drugs (lesser evil) and counseling to counter, overcome, cure the greater evil, addiction, drugs, alcohol, depression, anger, anxiety, etc. greater addiction to new drug(s). "Meet the new boss, same as the old boss."

Counseling: diet, herbs, exercise and spiritual practice (CH. 5, 29, 30) are the better choices for greater, more lasting, natural, drug-free happiness.

Has the past use of drugs or alcohol benefited, made you or anyone else a better person, truly happy, or done the opposite, depression, anxiety, laziness, sickness?

Aging

Function of time, sex (jing, ojas), diet, disease, climate, etc. Jing, ojas: reproductive, sexual essence ⇨

1. Fountain of youth: thick, colorful hair, moist, firm skin, greater energy, healing, etc. when full

2. Aging dryness, weakness, decline, physical and mental, when in decline

The following consume jing (CH. 4, 16) excessively:

1. Sex, orgasm: daily, weekly (3x). Less sex improves life, longevity. More info: CH. 5, 16.

2. Long-term low protein, fat diet consumes jing as replacement fuel. Animal flesh consumes more blood, nutrients, energy, jing to process.

3. Drugs, smoking, alcohol, insomnia, excessive exercise (especially when older)

Longevity:
- Vegetarian, dairy, organic, fruit, vegetables
- Whole grains (rice, wheat, oats), beans
- Almonds, walnuts, sesame seeds: raw, ground
- Smaller meals, fasting (1 day/ week) +/-
- "To lengthen thy life, lessen thy meals."
- Outdoor exercise, fresh air, sun bathing (20.min.)

AIDS, HIV

HIV (human immunodeficiency virus) attacks immune system ⇨ destroys lymphocytes, T cells ⇨ extreme ⇨ total breakdown ⇨ AIDS (Acquired Immune Deficiency Syndrome).

General symptoms (mild – severe):
- Bloating, gas, diarrhea, constipation
- Anemia, fatigue, pallor, weight loss, headaches
- Shortness of breath, poor circulation
- Pain (joints, muscles), inflammation, numbness
- Coughing, sore throat, mouth (lesions, sores)
- Thrush, swollen gums, glands, skin rashes
- Chronic fevers, restlessness, anxiety
- Insomnia, vertigo, palpitations, death

HIV infection rate: 20- 50%. Not everyone who is exposed develops HIV or AIDS. General causes:

1. Intravenous drug users, shared needles

2. Starvation, poor hygiene, or exposure to raw sewage (AIDS virus stays alive: 10- 11 days).

3. Incidence of AIDS:

a) Very low: lesbians (no ejaculation, lesser loss of essence), unlike heterosexual men (ejaculate), who generally have less sex than:

b) High: homosexuals via

- Excessive, daily sex, ejaculations, orgasms: reduces jing/ ojas ⇨ weakens health, immunity (CH. 4, 5, 16). Heterosexual generally less.

- Anal sex ⇨ bacteria ⇨ penis ⇨ blood ⇨ weaken immune system (AIDS, monkey pox), loosens anus, sphincter muscles ⇨ leaks jing, ojas

HIV, depending on health is curable. AIDS is more difficult, if curable (severity).

Treatment: CMD #1
- Milk (+ saffron) yogurt, ghee, whole grains, seeds (sesame), nuts (almonds), build ojas (CH. 5, 16)
- Chickpeas, cooked vegetables; turmeric
- Sarsaparilla: cleanses K, UB, sex organs

- Tonic herbs: American ginseng, saw palmetto, ashwagandha; marshmallow
- No sex
- + M. D.

Allergy (respiratory, food)

Abnormal, hypersensitive, allergic response to allergen (harmless or poisonous substance) ⇨

1. Respiratory:
- Pollen (ragweed), dog, cat hair, mold ⇨ lungs ⇨

General symptoms:
- Stuffy, runny nose, sinus, bronchial, congestion,
- Coughing, wheezing, sneezing, watery eyes
- Shortness of breath, chest tightness
- Swelling: tongue, throat difficulty swallowing
- Headache, fatigue, anaphylaxis

2. Diet, digestion via constitution (Ayurveda):
a) Vata: beans, corn, peanuts
b) Kapha: dairy, eggs, wheat, shellfish
c) Pitta: nightshades, tomatoes, potatoes, eggplant, peppers, sour fruit, peaches, strawberries

General symptoms:
- Intolerance, inability to digest certain foods
- Rash, hives, headache, fatigue
- Anaphylactic shock, death

3. Immune system response: mast cells (most tissues) ⇨ histamine (anti-inflammatory) ⇨
a) Widens small blood vessels ⇨ increases circulation, decreases blood pressure
b) Increases gastric secretions (stomach, HCl)

General causes:

1. Genetics (weak nervous system)

2. Diet, weak digestion, pasty, clogged intestines

Treatment: middle diet adjusted accordingly
- Stricter, organic vegetables (cooked > raw)
- Raw beets, peppermint tea: benefit lungs
- Avoid food, herbs ⇨ excess mucus, dryness
- Basil tea, honey: clears sinuses, phlegm
- Elimination of allergens; hay fever (CH. 22)
- + M.D.

3. Drugs, preservatives, penicillin, insects, mites
4. Chemicals (soaps, shampoos), liver disease, etc.

Alzheimer's Disease (presenile dementia)

Progressive decline, deterioration, drying of brain, nerves loss of mental function. Brain (nerves, 1/3 blood vessels): built, fueled, moistened, reddened by blood (nutrients). When autopsied the brains, cerebral arteries, neuro fibers of Alzheimer's patients were dry, brown, shrunken, tangled: blood deficiency, anemia.

General symptoms (starts ages 50- 60):
- Emotional instability, personality changes
- Memory lapses, disorientation, confusion, stupor
- Attacks women (low protein, fat diet, menstruation) 2x > men

General causes:

1. Diet

a) Deficient building, protein, fat (animal, plant)

Treatment: HMD
- Chicken, turkey, eggs, gotu kola, amla, guggul
- Ginkgo biloba increases circulation, blood ⇨ brain
- Avoid alcohol, drugs (destroy brain cells)
- +/- M.D.

b) Excess animal (> plant) sat. fat, cholesterol, protein ⇨ narrow, clogged arteries (chest, neck) ⇨ reduced blood flow ⇨ brain ⇨ dry, weak.

Treatment: CMD #1 + M.D.

2. Deficient jing (CH. 4, 16) dries, weakens brain

3. High levels: aluminum (deodorants, baking powder, processed foods, cookware), mercury

Amenorrhea

Abnormal stoppage or absence of menstrual flow.

General causes:

1. Excessive exercise ⇨ delay, stoppage

2. Diet: low protein fat ⇨ thin blood, anemia

Treatment: HMD
- Sesame seeds, amla, turmeric, myrrh
- +/- M.D.

3. Congenital abnormalities: reproductive tract

4. Endocrine, hormonal dysfunction, emotions

Anal Fissure

Small tear (papercut) in anus via straining, constipation, passing of hard or large stools ⇨
- Sharp pain during bowel movements +/- blood

General dietary cause:
- Overeating, excess protein, fat, oil, flour

Case History #26. Man (35): anal fissure via overeating, animal, fried foods, bread. His doctor told him: no cure, except operation, sew it back together, but: temporary incontinence (urine, bowels), impotence. I advised CMD, soft, watery grains (millet, rice), cooked vegetables, spices, etc. His fissure healed.

Anemia

Deficiency: red blood cells (RBC): low number or low RBC protein/ hemoglobin (high in iron, binds, transports oxygen) ⇨ decreases oxygen (body: 65%) ⇨
- Loss of appetite, constipation, headache
- Irritability, difficulty in concentrating
- Fatigue, weakness, cold extremities
- Pale lips, brittle nails, soreness in mouth
- Cessation of menstruation, loss of libido
- Pernicious anemia (vitamin B-12 deficiency)
- Hypoxia ⇨ tachycardia, shortness of breath, dizziness, fatigue, confusion

General causes:

1. Chronic illnesses, drugs, hormonal disorders

2. Repeated pregnancies, heavy menstrual bleeding

3. Lungs: excess mucus, asthma, pneumonia

4. Liver, thyroid disease, genetics, surgery, etc.

5. Diet: deficient building, protein, fat, vitamin B-12, iron, etc.

Treatment: HMD
- Animal (Vit. B-12), red meat, chicken, eggs, etc.
- Cooked vegetables (roots, sweet), beets, greens
- Almonds, sesame, flax seeds
- Amla, ashwagandha, ginseng, honey

Case history #27. Several women, vegan (ages 20-35): anemia (pale skin, diminished periods, thin hair, cracked nails). I advised animal (meat, chicken, turkey, eggs, dairy). Some took the advice and cured.

Treatment: CMD #1, 2
- Turmeric, yellow dock

Anger

Hot, fiery emotion. General causes:

1. Frustrated desire, inability to be calm, accept naturally occurring duality, never-ending alternating ups, downs, successes, failures of life.

2. Overeating animal, fried, spicy foods, alcohol ⇨ excess energy, pressure ⇨ explodes ⇨ anger

Treatment: CMD #1, smaller meals
• Chamomile, walking, meditation

Anxiety

Apprehension, excessive fear, worry, nervousness ⇨
• Rapid heartbeat, perspiration, panic attacks
• General causes: fear, diet, deficiency (jing, blood)

#8. Woman (65, vegetarian, S. Florida), strong, successful but frequent **anxiety** (fear, worry, nervousness, irritability, sweating), was screaming and yelling at me or her husband from one anxiety attack to another during consultation; incontinence (cannot hold urine), etc. My initial impression: excess heat, energy, however there was no excess fuel to create excess heat. She was suffering deficiency (blood, protein, fat) ⇨ weakness, lack of confidence, control but instead anxiety, fear, worry, for a person who was always strong, successful, positive. I recommended animal (meat, chicken, eggs), cooked vegetables, spices, etc. Problem: vegetarian. I told her it was a matter of life and death. She compromised, veal, eggs. Three days later, she called. I was a little nervous, thought I may have given her the wrong diet (too hot, animal, spices). When I answered, she asked, "Is this the genius?" She was very happy, no anxiety, having great bowel movements and teaching her employees deep abdominal breathing that I had taught her during consultation to calm her down.

Arteriosclerosis, atherosclerosis

Atherosclerosis (thickening, narrowing, hardening of arteries via plaque build-up in inner lining of artery.

General causes:
- High cholesterol, saturated fat, triglyceride
- High BP, smoking, diabetes, obesity, age

General symptoms:
- Chest pain, palpitations, shortness of breath
- Cold sweats, nausea, fatigue, dizziness, etc.

Arteriosclerosis (hardening via plaque build-up) ⇨
- Loss of elasticity ⇨ decreased blood flow especially to extremities: head, arms, legs ⇨
- Forgetfulness, confusion, difficulty talking
- Headaches, limping

General causes:
- Atherosclerosis, high cholesterol, saturated fat
- Processed, white flour: inorganic calcium ⇨ extreme ⇨ binds, dries, hardens arteries
- Excess sugar, fat (CH. 1) ⇨ triglycerides ⇨ thicken, harden arterial walls
- Smoking, old age

Treatment: CMD #1, 2
- Beets, celery, lettuce, leafy greens (raw or juice): high in nitrates: dilate, soften arteries
- Grains (barley, oats), nuts, seeds, beans: EFA
- Fruit (berries), juices (+ pulp), water (+++)
- Mild spices: cumin, coriander, fennel, turmeric
- Cayenne (clots), garlic, ginger: blood thinners
- More info: CH. 9 (Circulation)

Case history #4: I (53), overweight (20lb.), atherosclerosis, high blood pressure (150/120), changed ⇨ vegan, raw vegetables, fruit, juices, etc., 3 months ⇨ lost 20 lb., lowered BP: 110/70.

Arthritis

Generic term: musculoskeletal disease (inflammation of joint, bones, cartilage, ligaments, muscles, nerves) ⇨
- Pain (dull, sharp, migrating)
- Swollen, stiff, inflexible, numb, shake
- Dry, cracking sound: joints

Three major kinds:
1. Rheumatoid Arthritis: degeneration, atrophy of bones (CH. 20), women > men
2. Osteoarthritis: bone on bone, no cartilage (caps, cushions end of movable bones)
3. Gout (uric acid)

Addition arthritic type diseases:
- Restless Leg Syndrome (RLS), Psoriatic Arthritis
- Plantar Fasciitis (PF), Peripheral Artery Disease

The body, nerves, organs bones, ligaments, etc. are, built, fueled, moistened, cleansed, etc. by nutrients via blood.

General causes:

1. Anemia, thin, low protein, fat blood via low protein, fat diet ⇨ dry, weaken ⇨ arms, legs, nerves, muscles, etc. ⇨
- Rheumatoid arthritis, Plantar Fasciitis
- Restless Leg Syndrome, neuralgia

Treatment: HMD (no red meat)
- Vegetables, roots, round, greens, soups
- Hot spices: cinnamon, cayenne, ginger
- Ashwagandha, guggul, massage (sesame oil)

2. Excess saturated fat, cholesterol, protein ⇨
- Plaque, thick, narrow arteries (atherosclerosis), obesity ⇨ poor, reduced circulation, blood ⇨
- Legs ⇨ PF, RLS, Peripheral Artery Disease

3. Excess uric acid (animal, sugar, oatmeal) ⇨ blood, joints ⇨ crystallize ⇨ gout: needle shaped deposits ⇨ inflammation, jabbing pain: men (high animal) > women (low)

Treatment: CMD #1, 2
- Cooked vegetables, raw beets
- Apples, grapes, grapefruit break down uric acid
- Beets, celery, lettuce, leafy greens (raw or juice): high in nitrates (CH. 1); nuts, seeds, beans (EFA)
- Bitter herbs: guggul, aloe, turmeric, saffron
- Massage (sandalwood or coconut oil); ice pack

Case history #5. I (15- 54) arthritis, knee pain via basketball, diet (animal, white flour, etc.) and disease (narrow, clogged arteries). After a game I would be in severe pain, limp for several hours. In my 50's: three water on the knees (drained by M.D.). 54, stopped playing, changed my diet ⇨ CMD #1, more raw vegetables, grapes, juices ⇨ cured: no pain.

4. Excess soft dairy, sugar, fruit, juices, cold drinks ⇨ excess water, mucus, phlegm ⇨
- Swelling, edema, nodules ⇨ joints ⇨
- Dull heavy, aching pain, relieved by heat

Treatment: CMD #2
- Spices (cayenne, ginger, turmeric), guggul
- Mustard or turmeric compress (paste, add water)

5. Excess inorganic calcium via white flour: cookies, noodles, bread, chips, etc. ⇨ joints (hips, legs, knees, ankles) ⇨ pain: migrates ⇨ up, down

Treatment:
- Fruit, juice, beets (raw), eliminate white flour

Case history #25. I (68) vegan + animal crackers (white flour) +++ ⇨ pain. I stopped the crackers, increased raw (celery), cooked vegetables, grapes, grapefruit, cured in 2 weeks.

6. Sedentary lifestyle, injury

7. Diuretics (water pills) increase calcium excretion ⇨ fractures. **Case history #14**. Several elderly customers: bones (hands, feet) ⇨ thin, melted, fused or shattered (brother: lower leg).

8. Osteoarthritis: no dietary, herbal cure
•   Surgical gels (replace cartilage) injected ⇨ joints

9. Miscellaneous:

a) Tendonitis (pineapple), nerve pain (bayberry)

b) Ligaments: turmeric (internal or topical: paste)

c) Pain: massage (sandalwood or coconut oil)

d) Glucosamine sulfate (1500 mg/ day) via shellfish or bovine cartilage can grow cartilage only where there is some.

e) Manganese helps form cartilage, synovial fluids

f) Exercise. "A moving gate gathers no rust."

Asthma

Respiratory, lung disease:
•   Chronic mild to severe shortness of breath, cough, wheezing: dry or with phlegm
•   Breathing through the mouth, fast breathing
•   Tachycardia (fast heart rate), chest pain
•   Especially at night or during exercise
•   Anxiety, sleep apnea, early awakening, tiredness
•   Respiratory infections, hypoxia (deficient O_2)

General causes:

1. Drugs, allergies, kidney disease, genetics

2. Clogged lungs (excess water, mucus) via

a) Excess water, sugar, protein via dairy, juice, sodas, etc. ⇨ blood ⇨ lungs ⇨ water, mucus ⇨
- Alveoli ⇨ decreases oxygen absorption ⇨
- Rapid breathing (to increase oxygen intake), sleep apnea, hypoxia, etc.

b) Excess cold foods (ice cream, frozen yogurt), drinks (juice, water, sodas, etc.) ⇨
- Cool throat, chest ⇨ cools, slows, thickens water ⇨ lungs ⇨ mucus, phlegm (clear, white) ⇨
- Cough, shortness of breath etc.

Treatment: CMD #2
- Hot spices: cardamom, ginger, cayenne, etc.
- Bitters: mullein, sage, thyme, bayberry, turmeric (allergies), wild cherry bark
- Carrot juice, tangerine juice (decongestant)

3. Dry lungs via smoking, hot, dry climate

Treatment:
- Organic beets, lettuce, celery (raw or juice)
- Dairy, spices: fennel, cardamom
- Sour fruit juices: lemon, lime
- Ashwagandha, gotu kola, licorice, peppermint
- No smoking

Athlete's Foot

Fungal infection (ringworm) between toes ⇨ bacteria ⇨ infection, skin, turns white, itchy, cracks, peels off.

Topical treatments:
- Neem, tea tree oil, baking soda
- Soaking (foot, toes): apple cider vinegar

Attention Deficit Disorder (ADD)

Lack of focus, concentration generally applied to children or young adults. Blood, nutrients, reading, memory exercise, etc. strengthen the mind.

General causes:

1. Drugs, unstable home, boredom
2. Lack of attention, guidance (school, home)

3. Diet

a) Excess protein, fat ⇨ excess energy ⇨
- Nervousness, restlessness, poor concentration
- Treatment: CMD #1

b) Excess dairy dulls, slows the mind

c) Excess sugar (any) excites, irritates ⇨ restlessness, scattered attention

d) Deficient protein, fat (animal, plant) weakens the brain, decreases focus, attention
- Treatment: HMD

Case History #7. Mother, her daughter (11, pale, thin), not doing well in school, medically diagnosed: ADD, prescribed, taking **Adderall** and **Dexedrine** (stimulants, amphetamines*), which did not help. Her school (no M.D., psychiatrist) wanted to add **Ritalin** (*). Her mother was frustrated. Her daughter was not getting better. I asked if it was OK to question her daughter privately (some parents intimidate their kids)? Yes. I asked her daughter if her home was peaceful, loving? Yes. I believed her. Did she like red meat, chicken, vegetables (which ones), etc. to see if she would eat the diet, cure? Yes. I recommended the HMD, more personal attention. Six months later, I got a letter with report card (all A's, 1 B, math) thanking me.

Autoimmune Illnesses

Large group of diseases: abnormal immune system produces antibodies ⇨ attack normal tissues, fluids, etc.
- 80%: women (menstruation, low protein, fat diet)
- 20%: men (less deficient via high protein, fat)

Diseases:

1. Rheumatoid Arthritis (CH.19)
- Fatigue, low grade fever, loss of appetite
- Stiffness (A.M.), inflammation, swelling (joints)

2. Chronic Fatigue Syndrome (CH. 20)
- Extreme fatigue, aching muscles, joints
- Headaches, low blood pressure, fever
- Loose stools, diarrhea, constipation
- Candidiasis, depression, anxiety

3. Lupus
- Fatigue, abdominal pain, nausea, vomiting
- Diarrhea, constipation, weight loss, skin rash

4. Celiac disease: immune reaction to eating gluten
   (protein in wheat barley, rye)

5. Crohn's Disease (CH. 20)
- Abdominal pain: right side, appendix
- Diarrhea, nausea, fatigue, fever, weight loss

General causes:

1. Modern medicine: cause unknown
2. Chemical poisoning, bacteria, viruses
3. Chronic illness, genetics

4. Diet

a) Deficient protein, fat ⇨ extreme ⇨
- Anemia, low blood pressure, fatigue, dizziness
- Headaches, excessive weight loss
- Dry muscles, tendons, nerves
- Inflammation, swelling, stiffness, pain
- Constipation, cramps, depression, anxiety

Treatment: HMD (no red meat)
- Vegetables (cooked > raw), spices
- +/- M.D.

b) Excess protein, fat (red meat, chicken, turkey, fish, whole dairy), flour (bread, pretzels, crackers, chips, cookies), candy ⇨
- Pastes, clogs, ferments, inflames SI, LI ⇨
- Pain, reflux, acidity, nausea, colitis

c) Excess dairy, salads, fruit, juices, sodas, smoothies, cold drinks, sugar ⇨ extreme ⇨
- Indigestion, soft, hard abdominal bloating, pain
- Reflux, nausea, malabsorption, increased toxins
- Loose stools, excessive urination
- Mucus, phlegm, candidiasis, yeast (fungi)

Treatment: CMD #2
- Vegetables (cooked > raw)
- Hot spices, bitter herbs
- +/- M.D.

20. "B- C" DISEASES

Bleeding

1. Cuts, wounds

Treatment: topical
- Astringent (drying) herbs (red raspberry, self-heal, mullein, comfrey) stop bleeding
- Turmeric cream heals +/- prevents scarring

2. Minor nose bleeds (epistaxis)

Treatment:
- Yarrow (bitter, astringent): 3-5 drops (eyedropper)

3. Bleeding under skin (bluish, black spots) via

a) Injury, injections, viruses, tumors, fever

b) Arteries, veins (dry, fragile) via spicy, greasy, salty, acidic foods ⇨ thicken, dry, crack, bleed

Treatment: CMD #1
- Raw vegetables (beets, carrots, celery, lettuce)
- Hemostatic herbs: red raspberry (uterus), golden seal agrimony) cool the blood, stop bleeding
- Bitter herbs (blood cleansers): cold, drying

Body Odor

General causes:

1. Hygiene

2. Diet
a) Excess sugar (any): **sweet**
b) Dairy, alcohol, obesity: **sour**
c) Animal, fried foods: **foul**

d) Overeating ⇨ excessive digestion (fermentation, souring): **sour** breath (halitosis), body odor
e) Starvation diets, bulimia: **musty**

3. Diabetes (CH. 21): **sweet** odor, breath, urine

Treatment (dietary causes):
1. Sweet, sour body odor: CMD #2, spices
2. Foul body odor: CMD #1, bitter herbs
3. Musty body odor: HMD (no red meat, fish)
• Apple cider vinegar: underarm deodorant

It takes months of good diet, quality and smaller meals to cleanse, eliminate, replace old, stinky, diseased tissues, cells, fluids with new, healthy tissues, cells, etc.

Case history #28. I (60's, overweight) had sour body odor plus oily, hot rashes in both armpits via too much fat, sugar, candy, cookies, juices, etc. I changed my diet ⇨ CMD #2. Six months later ⇨ no sour smell and right rash (liver) cured, eliminated. The left (spleen) took 1½ years to cure. More info: CH. 25 (Rashes).

Bones

Protein, fat and jing are the substances, glue that holds minerals (calcium, magnesium, etc.), thickens, solidifies the bones, which thin naturally with age. The following weaken, thin or break the bones.

1. Decline in jing (CH. 16, Reproduction) via excessive sex, inactivity, old age, etc.

2. Gender: women, thinner, less dense bones, menopause (40's), decline in estrogen suffer osteoporosis (CH. 23) 80% >men (start age 65)

3. Pharmaceutical drugs: diuretics (water pills) increase calcium secretion ⇨ extreme (years) ⇨ decreases bone mineral density ⇨ fractures.

- My elderly customers (health food store) taking diuretics complained of bones dissolving, melting in their hands, feet. My brother's lower leg fractured while standing.

4. Diet

a) Long-term low protein, fat

b) Caffeine (coffee, colas, weight loss supplements, guarana): acidic ⇨ depletes, leaches calcium

c) Excess animal, sugar (any) stimulates pancreas ⇨ insulin ⇨ extracts calcium ⇨ excreted (urine)

Treatment: HMD (no red meat)
- Chicken, turkey, eggs, dairy
- Vegetables: cooked, especially green, leafy
- Nuts: almonds, walnuts (Omega-3), Brazil nuts: high calcium, magnesium, phosphorous
- Sesame seeds (black > white): organic unhulled, ground, 5- 10x more calcium > milk
- Seaweeds (high calcium), fish liver oil
- Ashwagandha: 5 grams/ day in milk; guggul
- Comfrey root, leaves; amla, Solomon's seal
- Avoid caffeine, concentrated sugars
- +/- M.D.

5. Sedentary lifestyle weakens the bones, muscles, etc. Exercise stimulates, strengthens, grows

Breast Disease

Breasts: watery, fatty tissue, lymph nodes.

1. Lumps, cysts (abnormal fluid filled sacs). Most breast lumps (common in childless women): harmless cysts: come and go.

2. Tumors (protein, fat), cancer (pure protein)

General causes:

1. Smoking, caffeine, hormones, menstrual cycle

2. Diet

a) Excess water, sugar, dairy, juices drinks ⇨ blood
    ⇨ soft, fatty breasts

Treatment: CMD #2
- Cooked vegetables, greens, radishes, kelp
- Turmeric, dandelion, golden seal root ⇨ reduce cysts, breast tumors; marshmallow (lumps)
- Spices: cayenne, black pepper, cardamom ⇨ coriander + corn silk, lemon grass: diuretic, reduces cysts
- Regular monitoring, self-examination
- +/- M.D.

b) Long-term high protein, sat. fat, cholesterol: red meat, chicken, turkey, fried foods, low fiber ⇨
- Breast tumor, cancer ⇨
- Firm, hard, immovable lump, malignant tumor
- Usually pain-free, swollen, or hot, inflamed, infected nipple: yellow, bloody, or clear discharge
- 12% women (age 40+)

Treatment: CMD #1, 2
- Organic vegetables red beets, lettuce, leafy greens (raw or juice): high nitrates, oxidizing enzymes detoxify body, kill cancer (anerobic)
- Shitake mushrooms, spices (no peppers)
- Essiac tea burdock, dandelion root, red clover
- Turmeric: stops precancerous, DNA changes
- +/- M.D.

Case history #2. Health food store. Two customers, women, age 60+ (past diet: red meat, chicken, fried foods, etc.) had cured their breast tumors, cancer via vegetarian diet and bitter herbs: Essiac tea by Marie Caisse, R.N. via native Indian medicine man (Canada).

Both had refused surgery and chemotherapy. Later, one started eating chicken. Her tumor came back. She stopped the chicken. The tumor disappeared within two months. Every disease, structure changes, builds up and breaks down via favorite (growth) and non-favorite (deterioration) foods, herbs, climates, etc.

"I have seen two **cancers of the breast** disappear with **fenugreek** seed in large amounts combined with a saltless vegetarian diet". "Max Gerson, M.D., **A Cancer Therapy, Results of Fifty Cases** (1958). **Dr. Albert Schweitzer** endorsed Max Gerson. "I see in Dr. Max Gerson one of the most eminent geniuses in medical history." Dr. Gerson also recommended **organic**.

3. Excess estrogen ⇨ growth in breasts, ovaries

General causes:
* Early menstruation (before age 9), obesity
* Late menopause (55), first child after age 40
* Stimulant drugs, estrogen supplements, soy

4. Underdeveloped breasts: saw palmetto berry
5. Mastitis: inflammation, pain, swelling: breast, lymph nodes (armpit) usually via bacterial infection or first two months of lactation

Treatment: marshmallow +/- M.D., antibiotics

Bronchitis

Inflammation of lungs, bronchi via

1. Smoking pastes, dries, irritates lungs, bronchitis

Treatment: dairy, honey, licorice, marshmallow
* More info: CH. 6 (Respiration); no smoking

2. Excess water, mucus, phlegm via excess protein, sugar, dairy, juices, smoothies, beer, soda, etc. ⇨ blood ⇨ lungs ⇨ cough, inflammation, cold, flu

Treatment: CMD #2
- Beans, cooked vegetables, mushrooms, turmeric
- Expectorants, diaphoretics (bayberry, cloves, ginger, licorice); anti-cough (gotu kola, mullein), pleurisy (bitter, pungent), myrrh
- Tangerine juice (decongestant), guggul, flaxseed
- +/- M.D.

3. Respiratory infection, virus, COPD, pollution

Cancer

Abnormal, uncontrollable growth of malignant (deadly) cells. Cancer cell: pure protein, anaerobic (grows without oxygen, dies in its presence) ⇨
- Kills normal cells
- Divide, grow uncontrollably into tumors
- Spreads (metastasize) ⇨ blood ⇨ body

General causes:

1. Toxins (poisons): smoking, pollution, household chemicals; plastic bottles, devitalized foods

2. Genetics, radiation, hormones (supplemental)

3. Diet: excess protein, saturated fat: red meat, chicken, turkey, butter, ice cream, etc. ⇨ tumors ⇨ benign (harmless) +/- deteriorate, ferment (bacteria) ⇨ cancer ⇨ all organs except heart (always pumping, moving)

Common cancers:

1. **Bladder** via fatty diet, smoking, toxins, etc. ⇨
- Painful, burning, frequent urination + blood

2. **Breast** via diet, caffeine smoking, poisons, emotions ⇨
- #2 cause of cancer, death: women. Lungs (#1).
- More info: CH. 20, Breast Disease, case history

3. **Cervical** via infection: sex (human papilloma virus/ HPV), fatty diet, poisons ⇨ hard to detect, usually no symptoms until advanced ⇨
- Bleeding: douching, intercourse, between periods

4. **Colorectal** via diet, weak digestion, poisons ⇨
- Rectum: blood in stools (tumors bleed)
- Alternating constipation, diarrhea, bloating, pain
- Anemia, significant weight loss, death (#2: cancer)

5. **Esophageal** via diet, smoking
- Hard to diagnose until advanced ⇨
- Dysphagia (difficulty swallowing), vomiting (blood)

6. **Laryngeal** (throat) via smoking, chemical poisons: diet, pollution, etc. ⇨
- Persistent cough, sore throat, ear pain

7. **Leukemia** via toxins, poisons: diet, pollution, etc.) ⇨ blood ⇨ lymph system, spleen, bones ⇨
- Pallor, fatigue, shortness of breath, weight loss
- Excessive sweating, easily bruising, nose bleeds
- Swollen lymph nodes, enlarged spleen, liver

8. **Lung** (CH. 6) via smoking, diet, chemical poisons, pollution ⇨
- Persistent cough (+/- blood), shortness of breath
- Chest pain, fatigue, weight loss
- Recurring bronchitis, pneumonia

9. **Lymphoma** via toxins, poisons ⇨
- Lymph system/ nodes ⇨
- Shortened breath, nausea, vomiting, headaches
- Abdominal bloating, seizures (nodes in head)

10. **Pancreas** via diet ⇨
- Pancreatitis (CH. 24), nausea, vomiting
- Severe pain (burning, stabbing): back (left side), upper abdomen (+ swelling), around navel
- See following case history

11. **Prostate** (CH. 24) via diet, sex, withholding of orgasm, ejaculation (CH. 16)

12. **Skin** via diet, smoking, radiation, overexposure to sun, especially fair skinned people ⇨
- Growths, lumps: nose, neck, ears ⇨
- Ulcerated, change color (dark, purple), bleed, scabs (come, go)

- **Melanoma**: tumors under skin. My brother, ex-smoker (30 years): Stage 3 melanoma: left side of body below arm-pit (no sun exposure), surgically removed, cured, never returned.

13. **Stomach** via diet: overeating, excess animal (flesh), spicy, sour, fried foods, sugar, alcohol, coffee, smoking ⇨
- Indigestion, pain, bloating, vomiting after eating
- Stomach pain that does not go away

14. **Testicular** men 20- 35 via diet, sex ⇨
- Lump(s), enlarged testicle, thickened scrotum
- Blood in semen
- Breast enlargement

Treatment: CMD #1, 2
- Milk, ghee
- Organic vegetables, raw or juiced beets (anti-tumor), lettuce, leafy greens (nitrates, oxygen)
- Bitters: red clover (skin, breasts, ovaries), dandelion, burdock root, myrrh, turmeric, barberry: digest protein, fat, anti-inflammatory/ septic/ tumor/ cancer
- Selenium (anti-tumor: lungs, colon, prostate)
- Oxygen therapies: ozone (too much: harm, kill); food grade hydrogen peroxide: 2- 3 drops in 3C water, empty stomach, 1- 2x/ day, 3x/ week. Too much ⇨ bleeding (throat, stomach).
- Daily exercise, fresh air
- Reduce, eliminate sex
- +/- M.D., drugs, surgery, etc.

Case history #29. Jean Kohler, professor of music (Ball State University, IN): **pancreatic cancer** (1973) given one month to live, tried, stopped chemotherapy, went to Boston: Michio Kushi ⇨ strict macrobiotic, vegan diet, no fish ⇨ **6 months** ⇨ cured. Most doctors were skeptical. 8 yrs. later died undergoing exploratory surgery (found traces of pancreatic cancer). **Cancer Prevention Diet** by Michio Kushi, Alex Jack

Cancer is anaerobic, dies in the presence of oxygen.

"It is known in **primitive forms** of life the **energy** of the **cells** is derived from almost entirely from **anaerobic** conditions or through **fermentation**. In **higher** animals the **lower** fermentative anaerobic systems are mixed with **oxidation systems**, whereby more molecular **oxygen** is utilized, transported from the respiration of the lungs. **The malignancies** in human beings continuously fall back deeper and deeper into **fermentation**. The major part of the **body** becomes more **poisoned** and more **reduced** in its defense and healing power. The ideal task of **cancer therapy** is to restore the function of **oxidizing systems**. In the entire organism, this of course is difficult to accomplish. It involves the following: detoxifying of whole body, increasing **potassium** (fruit, vegetables), oxidizing enzymes daily. **A Cancer Therapy** by Max. Gerson. M.D.

Beets (raw or juice): high nitrates, increase circulation, oxygen; tumor inhibiting, anti-cancerous.

"One of the most remarkable and tremendously successful programs for treating many kinds of **cancer tumors** was commenced in the late 1950's by Alexander Ferenczi M.D., Department of Internal Diseases, district hospital, Csoma, Hungary using only **raw red beets**... In D.S. a man 50 years of age, lung tumor was diagnosed by me, confirmed in a Budapest hospital: **lung cancer**. I started the treatment in the prescribed manner. After six months the tumor disappeared." He also successfully treated **prostate** cancer with beetroot.

"When admitted, he was bedridden with a permanent catheter. After 1 month (beets) the catheter was removed. The patient walked around." **Heinerman's New Encyclopedia of Fruits & Vegetables**, p. 39

Visualization mind over matter.

(1) News report: young child cured, eliminated his brain tumor by visualizing Star Wars, space ships shooting deadly rays to destroy his tumor, little by little.

(2) Medical journal (Europe): schizophrenic patient, multiple personalities, one: diabetic, needed insulin except when reverted to another personality that did not diagnose, test positive (diabetes), require insulin.

Chemotherapy poisons, kills healthy and unhealthy issues. Vegetable soups (seaweed, spices); salt, seaweed baths help eliminate toxins, radiation.

Candidiasis

Yeast-like infection via abnormal growth of Candida (normal fungus/ yeast in large intestine) ⇨ blood ⇨

- Indigestion, bloating, gas, acidity, food allergies
- Chronic low-grade fevers, fatigue, weakness
- Fever, thirst, acute infections
- Loss of taste, pain swallowing, eating
- Cracking, redness (corners of mouth
- Oral thrush, white patches
- Lesions (tongue, inner cheek)
- Skin: rash between toes, fingers
- Vagina: itchy yeast infection, white discharge
- Attacks women more than men

General causes:

1. Weak immunity, medications, antibiotics
2. Hormonal changes, diabetes poor hygiene
3. Climate (cold, hot, damp)

4. Weak digestion (common: vata, kapha constitutions, diets) ⇨ increased waste, poisons ⇨ LI ⇨ destroys normal bacterial balance ⇨ Candida

5. Diet

a) Vata, deficient protein, fat, excess salads, fruit, juices) ⇨ thin blood, anemia ⇨ #1- 4, insomnia

Treatment: CMD #2, chicken, turkey
- Whole grains, hot spices (garlic, basil, cayenne)
- Avoid meat, dairy (except buttermilk, ghee), gaseous vegetables, salads, beans, sweet fruits, juices, sugars, yeast

b) Kapha: excess sugar (any), soft dairy, fruit, juices, smoothies, beer, etc. ⇨ blood ⇨ #1- 6

Treatment: CMD #2
- Grains (rye, corn, millet), beans (mung)
- Hot spices: ginger, cardamom, pau d'arco tea
- Bitters: chamomile, golden seal, barberry root
- Avoid sugar, salads, dairy, etc.

c) Excess protein, fat ⇨ #1, 4- 6

Treatment: CMD #1
- Raw foods, greens, chlorophyll juice
- Spices, bitters (golden seal, barberry, gentian)
- Pau D'arco tea

Cellulite

Excess water, fat accumulates ⇨ pockets (abdomen, thighs): women (dominated by water) > men (fire) via dairy, salads, cold drinks, juices, sodas, etc.

Treatment: HMD (no red meat, fish) or CMD #2
- Cooked vegetables, beans, hot spices
- Bitters (golden seal, gentian, aloe vera, barberry) 1- 2x/day. Too much weakens digestion.

Case history #11. Woman (35, trim), cold, damp, sweet diet ⇨ cellulite ⇨ reduced via CMD #2, bitters.

Chronic Fatigue Syndrome

General symptoms (six months, life-time)
- Extreme fatigue, loss of appetite, headaches
- Aching muscles, inflamed joints, fever
- Constipation, loose stools, diarrhea
- Mucus, phlegm, viral infections, Candidiasis
- Women (menstruation, anemic diet) more than men

General causes:
- Viral infection, immune system dysfunction
- Hormonal imbalances, insomnia, diet, etc.
- More info: Autoimmune (CH. 19)

Cirrhosis

Hardening of liver tissue into fiber, lobules ⇨
- Fatigue, nausea, vomiting, cramps, itching
- General causes: alcoholism, fatty diet, etc.

Treatment: M.D. +
- Vegetables, raw beets, green juices, gotu kola

Cold, Flu

Respiratory viruses (common cold, flu) **thrive** in stagnant fluids (water, mucus, etc.), deficiency, obesity.

1. **Common cold** (less serious)
- Coughing, mucus, stiff shoulders, shaking
- Sore throat, swollen glands, fever

Treatment:
1. **Starve a cold**: eliminate cold foods, drinks, (dairy, sugar, juices, sodas, etc.), mucus:
- Bitter herbs: cold, drying, antiviral, antiseptic:
- Golden seal, echinacea combination
- Yellow dock cleanses swollen glands

2. **Feed a fever**: increase body temperature ⇨ burns, eliminates mucus, kills viruses via
- Hot spices (vegetables, soups, teas):
- Cardamom, ginger, licorice: sore throat
- Basil: diaphoretic (sweating), reduces mucus
- Garlic expectorant (eliminates mucus, phlegm), disinfectant, cleanses blood, lymph glands, lymph
- Peppermint heats, dissolves mucus, phlegm opens the lungs, improves digestion
- Sage (pungent, bitter): diaphoretic, expectorant, sore throat, laryngitis, swollen lymph glands
- Hot bath: cover quickly after to avoid cold draft ⇨ re-infect

Common cold: generally curable at the onset, day 1, 2 via diet, herbs, if healthy, in good shape, lean.

Case history #19. At a pool with friend (30's, athlete) who was coughing non-stop, every five minutes. He said it was his allergies. I said it was a cold that he needed to eat hot foods. He held up his beer. I told him he needed spices, which he did not like. Too bad. I went into his mother's kitchen, used every spice I could find and made him a dragon hot vegetable soup. He gobbled down two bowls. 20 minutes later, no cough or runny nose.

II. **Flu** (severe cold) ⇨
- Coughing, swollen glands tonsillitis (strep), fever
- Difficulty breathing, loss of taste (COVID), death

U.S.A. (330 million): 40% vaccinated/ year
- 10% (33 million) mostly unvaccinated catch the flu: mild, low death rate until COVID.

Treatment: 7 days +/- to cure if healthy
- CMD #1 (vata, thin)
- CMD #2 (kapha, obese)
- Peppermint tea, bitters, golden seal (tonsillitis)
- Tea: 1 TB licorice (simmer 5 min.) + ½ tsp. each: ginger, cardamom (loss of taste) 2x/ day
- +/- M.D., antibiotics

<u>2020</u>: COVID, no vaccine, except normal flu
- 30 million sick (9%), 400,000 deaths (1.3%)
- #3 (death): majority: obese, heart disease *
- 60% unvaccinated: did not get sick or report

<u>2021</u>: COVID vaccine: same numbers

<u>2022</u>: COVID (60% vaccinated): 30 million (9%) sick (mostly unvaccinated), 300,000 deaths *

World (8 billion): 250 million COVID cases/ yr. = 3%

U.S.A. despite "best" doctors, technology, shutdown, isolation: #1: COVID infections, deaths.

Best prevention, most flu resistant, quickest curing: young, healthy, lean or active.

Flu vaccine: generally safe, effective, short-term (4-6 months) answer, cure, protection. It does not change diet nor strengthen immunity long-term. Occasional sickness does, just as daily exercise strengthens the bones, muscles, locomotion, while inactivity weakens.

Constipation

Normal bowel movement: 2x daily, if eating two to three meals per day, prevents reabsorption of toxins back into bloodstream (autointoxication). Constipation: Infrequent or difficult elimination ⇨ retention of stools ⇨
- Cramping, bloating, pain
- Nausea: relieved by bowel movement
- Autoimmune, tumors, cancer

General causes:

1. Diet
a) Excess protein, fat, sugar, flour ⇨
- Pastes, dries, hardens SI, LI
- Hard, painful bloating, dry, hard stools
- Mild constipation, diverticulosis/itis, cancer

Treatment: CMD #1
- Prune or grape juice upon rising, water (++)
- Fruit for breakfast. Avoid coffee on empty stomach (dries, weakens ST, descending energy)
- Raw > cooked vegetables, spacing meals

Pain occurs as paste dislodges and intestinal walls regain their moisture, elasticity

b) Deficient protein, fat, vegetables, fruit ⇨
- Dry stools, severe constipation

Treatment: HMD, CMD #1
- Oily foods (dairy, nuts), whole grains (oats)
- Cooked vegetables + olive or sesame oil 2x/ day
- Ginger, cardamom, fennel (bloating, gas)
- Severe constipation: aloe vera gel or senna, rhubarb: 2 days. Avoid: diarrhea, hemorrhoids, inflammation, stones, pregnant, lactating.
- +/- M.D.

c) Excess dairy, salads, juices, cold drinks ⇨
- Mild constipation, stools (white, copious, phlegm)

Treatment: CMD #2
- Spices, bitter herbs; flax seeds: soaked or ground

2. Excess bitter herbs, diuretics, laxatives; coffee, smoking, sex (CH. 16), enemas, colonics ⇨ extreme drains energy, dries, weakens LI

3. Old age (less energy, activity), drugs

4. Sedentary life-style ⇨ mild constipation

Cough

General causes:

1. Cold foods, drinks, juices, sugar, dairy, etc. ⇨
- Water, mucus ⇨ LG ⇨ wet cough, expectoration

Treatment: CMD #2
- Cooked, gaseous vegetables
- Spices, bitter herbs

2. Deficient protein, fat, excess spices, bitters
3. Smoking, extreme hot, dry, windy climate ⇨
- Dry lungs, throat, cough

Treatment: CMD #1
- Milk, honey

Case history #18. I (60): dry cough, all night long, five days. Diet: dry, vegan (low protein, fat), spices, bitter herbs, coffee. I added milk, eggs, walnuts, more cooked vegetables, decreased hot spices, eliminated bitters ⇨ 3 days, cured.

Crohn's Disease

Chronic inflammatory condition: large or small intestine (end) ⇨
- Fever, weight loss, fatigue
- Abdominal pain, nausea, diarrhea, constipation
- Inflammation, ulcerative colitis, Crohn's

General causes:

1. Food allergies, bacterial infections, antibiotics

2. Diet: excess meat, eggs, dairy, fat, flour, juices, sugar, soda, candy ⇨ paste, clog, ferment, inflame SI, LI ⇨ pain, nausea, diarrhea, etc.

Treatment: CMD #2
- +/- M.D.

Case history #30. 1985, Mother came into store with son (13): Crohn's. His diet: dairy, juice, soda, sugar, etc. I advised CMD #2, spices +/- chicken, turkey. He cured.

21. "D- F" DISEASES

Depression

Depression: unhappy, dull, negative state of mind, reaction to life, body, aging, disease, society, etc. ⇨
- Dejection, feeling of worthlessness
- Chronically sad, angry; lazy
- withdrawal, antisocial, suicidal thoughts
- Women more than men

Two kinds:

1. Normal: **unipolar** (occasional depression)

2. Abnormal: **bipolar** (2- 4% adults): frequent, daily, weekly, alternates hyperactivity, talking, elation, violence ⇔ isolation, depression, mania (delirium), little or no control

General causes:

1. Age, energy, health
- Happy: young, active, healthy, energetic
- Depressed: older, lesser energy, health, activity, greater disease, pain, isolation, boredom

2. Chemical imbalance, low levels of serotonin (neurotransmitter): relaxes, eases tension, calms the mind. Poultry, eggs, milk, nuts, seeds: high tryptophan (amino acid produces serotonin)

3. Gender: women more susceptible via
- Hormonal changes
- Deficiency (menstruation, low protein, fat diet)
- Patriarchal society, religion than
- Men: opposite (hot, angry) via excess energy, testosterone, high animal, alcohol, power, etc.

- U.S.A., many countries, religions (East, West) fiercely patriarchal (male dominated): endless misogyny, violence, dehumanizing abuse, 2nd class, servile treatment: women; minorities, etc.

4. Life, society: patriarchy, violence, greed, ignorance, inequality, wars, pollution: depressing

5. Television, movies, video games, etc. excite, dull, indoctrinate, train, addict the mind to endless "normal" pleasures and excitement of violence, sex, greed, power, etc. ⇨ depression, anger

6. Sex (CH. 16), drugs (all), alcohol

7. Climate:
- Fall, winter (cold, damp, dark) ⇨ less energy, stimulation ⇨ greater inactivity ⇨ depression
- Spring, summer (hot, sunny, light) ⇨ greater energy, stimulation, activity ⇨ happiness

8. Mind (thinks, chooses, reacts, directs energy) ⇨ depression, anger, etc. or happiness, peace.

Depression (lack of happiness): natural, normal reaction to life, when happiness (cure) = body, youth, family, friends, job, possessions, etc. ⇨ age, decline, bore or end with time ⇨ disappoint, sadden.

Depression anger, right, wrong, success, failure, good, bad, etc. ⇨ **taught** ⇨ experts: family, friends, society, politicians, priests, M.D.s, internet who are not always right, expert, correct, and sometimes wrong.

Depression is more common in the West (material) than East (spiritual), which places more importance on God. Happiness is the cure.

Part-time happiness is the best the mind can do when attached to anything finite, unlike the spirit: infinite and forever joyous. Life is body, mind and spirit (Spirit).

9. Spirit (God)

Ayurveda (Hinduism), Chinese Medicine (Taoism, Buddhism) ⇨ **spirit** ⇨ gateway to lasting happiness and supernatural powers via the Greater Spirit via:

Seven chakras, spiritual energy centers (brain, spine), structures, functions ⇨ divine, supernatural ⇨
- Powers (control of energy, matter)
- Pleasures, never-ending peace, joy, etc. via:

Spiritual practice (CH. 29, 30), especially:

a) Meditation (CH, 30), thoughts, actions change the brain (vinyl album, thought grooves) for better ⇨ neuroplasticity: eliminates old, negative grooves, thoughts, memories, replaces with new, positive, spiritual thoughts, grooves. Replaying negative thoughts, people, events deepen those grooves.

b) Kindness, generosity. It always feels good to do good, despite "no good deed goes unpunished."

c) Good company. "Be always with people who inspire you; surround yourself with people who lift you up. Do not let your resolutions and positive thinking be poisoned by bad company. Even if you cannot find good company to inspire you, you can find it in meditation." Paramahansa Yogananda, **Journey to Self-Realization**, p. 370

d) Inspirational books, words, lives of Jesus, Krishna, Buddha, Lao Tzu, Moses, true saints present, past (men, women) of all true religions: walked on water, healed the sick, raised the dead, etc., remained forever joyous, humble, charitable, loving, despite disease, pain, homelessness, persecution. More info: **Mystics and Miracles** Bert Ghezzi.

e) Choose your own hero(es), lasting inspiration.

f)   Solitude, privacy to concentrate on the solution, escape bad influences, people, environments

g)   Outdoor exercise, walking, fresh air, trees to relax the mind, replace and stop depressing thoughts.

"To do is to know. To know is to do."

Spiritual powers and pleasures are theoretical promises, until realized, personally experienced. Other people's experiences, truths are nice, but no substitute for one's own spiritual practice, vision.

Modern medicine treats depression with stimulant drugs (amphetamines) that may temporarily work, give a solution, new "high" but also

1.   Damage the brain, nerves, weaken will power and clear thinking necessary to overcome depression

2.   Numb, high the mind, divert attention away from depressing thoughts, until "high" wears off ⇨
•   Greater craving, addiction, depression, mania, as they do not remove the cause.

Recreational drugs: no different, may temporarily help, but also harm, addict, weaken.

Counseling, new friends, jobs, cosmetic surgery, etc. temporarily help, inspire but do not guarantee lasting happiness. Spiritual practice (+/- belief in God) is the only way to not only achieve bliss, but also find out who, what the spirit, God really is.

Detoxification

Detoxification cleanses, eliminates cholesterol, drugs, poisons, metals, etc., depending on severity. Withdrawal, cleansing symptoms, pain (physical, mental) occurs but lessens with time. Too much detoxing or radical dietary changes can also harm.

General ways to detox:

1. Vegetarian diet, **organically grown** produce, herbs. Non-commercial: generally high artificial fertilizers, preservatives, dyes, insecticides, etc. Changing from meat, fish, etc. to vegetarian diet is radical: requires transition.

2. Vegetables, raw (beets, greens, lettuce: nitrates, circulation, oxygen), fruit: cleanses LV, SI, LI

3. Yams, sweet potatoes help eliminate metals

4. Spices (digestion, anti-septic/ inflammatory/ viral., etc.), digestive enzymes (supplements) Avoid excessive use ⇨ weakens digestion

5. Smaller, earlier, spaced meals (4 hrs.): easier to digest, cleanse, eliminate (CH. 7, Digestion)

6. Bitter herbs (CH. 3):
• Antibiotic, antibacterial, antiviral, laxative, etc.
• Cleanse, thin the blood
• Increase beneficia digestive bacteria (flora)
• Avoid if thin, dry, weak, blood thinners, pregnant

7. Milk Thistle: reduces toxins in the liver

8. Psyllium husks (absorb water), clay (minerals) cleanses the intestines; but also destroys flora (acidophilus, probiotics help restore)
• Contraindicated: edema, cellulite, yeast, Candidiasis, emaciation, autoimmune illness

9. Fasting: fruit, juice, herbs, water if strong.
• One to three days/ week, 1x/ month if strong. Check with your doctor.
• Start, end fast light: vegetable soups, broth or disastrous results may occur: About the Author.
• Relaxes, cleanses, strengthens: ST, SI, LI, LV
• Contraindicated: cold, thin, dry, deficient, weak

10. Exercise increases circulation, elimination, body temperature, helps kill bacteria, viruses, eliminate toxins, drugs via skin. Walking in nature increases oxygen (purifies blood, anti-cancer), circulation, elimination. Avoid excessive exercise if weak or chronically ill. Ask M.D.

Detoxing: cleanses, drains energy, releases poisons ⇨ extreme ⇨ sicken

a) Best times: spring, summer (excess energy, heat) generally require less building, energy

b) Worst: fall, winter (cold) or if thin, weak, sick, cold increases susceptibility to colds, flu

Drugs, tobacco, marijuana, poisons, heavy metals, etc. take time (months, years) to detox, if not too severe. The longer or deeper the toxin (brain, nerves, bones, etc.), the longer, more painful the detox. Consult an M.D. If you do not eat, you do not have to detox it.

Diabetes Mellitus

Metabolic, blood sugar (body's main energy source) disorder (high, low) via pancreas, liver, kidneys (anti-diuretic hormone/ ADH), pituitary gland (ADH), lack or failure of insulin to transport glucose into cells, but instead collects in blood.

Pancreas (lower left side behind stomach) produces hormones (CH. 8) ⇨ regulate blood sugar (glucose):

1. **Insulin** transports glucose ⇨ cells
• Excess glucose ⇨ glycogen (stored liver, muscles)

2. **Glucagon** converts glycogen (stored in liver) ⇨ glucose ⇨ bloodstream ⇨ raises blood sugar

Kidneys filter the blood, remove poisons, nitrogen, excess water, glucose, etc. ⇨ urine ⇨ urination.

General symptoms:

- Hyperglycemia (high blood sugar)

- Fatigue, hunger (lack of usable energy/ glucose not entering cells), weight loss, confusion

- Excessive urine (sweet odor), urination, fluid loss ⇨ dehydration ⇨ thirst, dry mouth via excess blood sugar ⇨ overworks the kidneys, filter ⇨ draws more water ⇨ increases urine, urination.

- Slow-healing wounds, sores (sugar dissolves)

- Frequent infections. Excess sugar feeds bacteria (urinary tract), yeast (genital, oral areas).

- Blurred vision, seeing dark spots (floaters)

- Acanthosis nigricans (AN): dry, itchy skin, dark velvety skin patches, skin tags

- Diabetic neuropathy: damage (excess glucose) to peripheral nerves: feet, hands ⇨ numbness, cramps, burning, tingling pain, muscle weakness

- Brain fog, confusion, stupor

Two types:

1. Type 1: **juvenile** (genetic) or young adult
- Autoimmune disease: immune system destroys cells that produce insulin ⇨ hyperglycemia
- Requires insulin, diet, herbs, managed only
- Excess insulin, missed meals, excess exercise ⇨ hypoglycemia (too little blood sugar)

2. Type 2: **adult onset**
- Pancreas: little or no insulin ⇨ high blood sugar
- Insulin resistance: body does use insulin properly

General causes:

1. Obesity, physical inactivity, disease

2. Diet

a) Excess sugar (natural, synthetic), high glycemic foods (CH. 8, Blood Sugar): white bread, rice, pasta, watermelon, cream of wheat, instant oatmeal, corn flakes, pancakes, processed snacks (doughnuts, chips, crackers, cookies, etc.)

b) Coffee raises blood sugar ⇨ overworks pancreas

c) Excess saturated fat, cholesterol: red meat, pork, chicken, turkey, fish, whole dairy, fried foods ⇨
- Excessive belly fat around abdominal organs ⇨
- Insulin resistance (cells do not respond to insulin)

Treatment: CMD #1, 2

Low glycemic foods (0- 55): raise blood slowly
- Fruit: apples, berries, oranges, pears, bananas. Raisins help stabilize blood sugar
- Vegetables: broccoli, cauliflower, tomatoes spinach, carrots, sweet potatoes, yams, hard squash, parsnips. Raw celery leaves (insulin).
- Grain (complex sugar raises blood sugar slowly): barley, bulgur, bran, whole wheat, oats, quinoa, brown rice
- Beans (lowers blood sugar*): lentils, chickpeas, kidneys, adukis, etc.
- Nuts, seeds: almonds, cashews, sesame, etc.
- Dairy (lactose): low-fat milk, yogurt, cheese
- Non-carbohydrates: meat, poultry, fish eggs, fats, oils, herbs: zero GI
- Hot spices (black pepper, cayenne, ginger, etc.) help reduce blood glucose levels
- Bitters (berberine): golden seal, barberry, dandelion root, guggul, gymena sylvestre; turmeric (1- 3 grams 2- 3x/day with aloe gel) *.

- Caution: long-term use (all bitters) weakens the pancreas, all function. Avoid if weak, thin, cold.

- +/- M.D.

Case history #31. Friend (72) **diabetes mellitus** diagnosed (40's) cured (no insulin, 20 years) via diet, bitter herbs and apple cider vinegar. However, he still suffers from high blood sugar, as he has not been able to perfect his diet, forcing him to constantly monitor, control his blood sugar via herbs.

Long-term diabetes mellitus ⇨
- Fatigue, insomnia, excessive weight loss
- Wasting away of tissues, burning (hands)

Treatment: HMD
- Beef broth, dairy, ghee
- Whole grains, nuts, sweet vegetables
- Turmeric, gymena sylvestre, ashwagandha
- +/- M.D.

Diarrhea

Frequent loose, watery stools (+/- blood, mucus) ⇨
- Abdominal bloating, cramps
- Decreased nutrient absorption
- Fatigue, weakness, dehydration
- Death

General causes:
1. Spoiled foods, bacteria, parasites, viruses
2. Drugs, antibiotics, contaminated water
3. IBS, ulcerative colitis, Crohn's

4. Diet

a) Excess fat, oil, sugar, cold foods
b) Bad food combinations (milk + meat or fish) ⇨
- Diarrhea, yellow, foul smelling (+/- blood, pus)
- Burning sensation (rectum, anus), fever

Treatment: CMD #1
- Light diet: cooked vegetables, whole grains
- Bitters: golden seal, barberry, senna (onset)
- Astringent (red raspberry leaf), nutmeg
- +/- M.D.

c) Excess soft dairy, sugar, juices, cold drinks ⇨
- Diarrhea, white, more quantity, infrequent

Treatment: CMD #2
- Light diet, dried ginger, cayenne, black pepper
- +/- M.D.

5. Amoebic dysentery via poor sanitation

Treatment
- Garlic, wormwood, hot spices +/- M.D.

6. Infantile diarrhea via inability to digest milk

Treatment:
- Spices: cardamom, fennel, dill help digest dairy
- Mother ⇨ blood ⇨ breast milk
- Small amounts in baby's milk
- + M.D.

Dizziness

Nervous disorder via sudden interruption, decrease in blood (oxygen, protein, etc.) ⇨ brain ⇨ dizziness, swaying, loss of consciousness.

General causes:

1. Diet:

a) Excess protein, saturated fat, cholesterol thicken, narrow ⇨ coronary arteries ⇨ decreased blood, oxygen ⇨ brain ⇨ dizziness on exertion

b) Deficient protein, fat dries, weakens the brain

2. Dehydration, hypoglycemia, migraine

3. Motion sickness, inner ear problems, drugs

4. Smoking (tobacco, marijuana), anxiety, stress

5. Insomnia (CH. 23), M.S., Alzheimer's (CH. 19)

Dysmenorrhea

Painful, difficult menstruation before and during period. Symptoms vary according to diet (CH. 16) and constitutional tendencies (CH. 5, Ayurveda).

1. Vata (air) constitution
2. Deficient protein, fat ⇨
• Deficient hormones, fluids
• Dry uterus ⇨ cramps; dry skin,
• Constipation, palpitations, anxiety

Treatment: HMD
• Chicken, turkey, eggs, cooked vegetables
• Ginger, nutmeg, turmeric
• Licorice (moistening), Evening primrose oil
• Valerian (cramps, relaxant), chamomile
• Massage lower abdomen: warm sesame oil (or douche)
• +/- M.D.

3. Pitta (fire) constitution
4. Excess protein, fat, cholesterol, salt, spices, fermented foods, drinks, etc.⇨
• Burning, loose stools, diarrhea
• Thicker blood, clots, tumors ⇨ uterus ⇨ dysmenorrhea, endometriosis

Treatment: CMD #1
• Mold spices: cumin, coriander, fennel
• Bitters: skullcap, hops, gotu kola, myrrh
• +/- M.D.

5. Kapha (water) constitution
6. Excess dairy, juice, sugar, cold drinks ⇨ uterus ⇨
• Dysmenorrhea, vaginal discharge
• Kapha (water)

Treatment: CMD #2
• Grains, beans, cooked vegetables
• Spices: ginger, cinnamon, nutmeg, turmeric, cumin, coriander, fennel
• Bitters: aloe vera, valerian, gotu kola, skullcap, myrrh (cleanses uterus)
• +/- M.D.

Eczema

Inflammatory skin condition:
• Thin, dry, cracked, itching, bleeding skin
• Blister like formations ⇨ weep, release fluid, pus before forming a crust ⇨ scale, flake, spread

General causes:

1. Food allergies, Candidiasis

2. Diet

a) Deficient protein, fat thins, dries, cracks the skin

b) Excess salads, fruit, sugar, sodas, ice water ⇨
• Dilute, decrease digestion, absorption, thin the blood, increase poisons ⇨
• Thin, weaken, infect: skin

Treatment: HMD, no red meat, fish
• Chicken, turkey, seeds, nuts, spices
• Echinacea, gotu kola, golden seal, neem

Case history #23. 1989, I (macrobiotic diet, 10 years, mostly vegan low protein, fat, salads, fruit, juices, sugar) living in South Florida: bad case of **eczema**.

It started as one blister (left index finger) ⇨ months ⇨ all fingers multiple blisters, cracked skin, pus, bleeding ⇨ back of hand ⇨ arm ⇨ right hand, fingers. It was gross. I had to wear surgical gloves in the store and at school, where some thought it was herpes. I then rubbed my fingers, blood on my face. Nothing happened. It was not herpes. I tried every Chinese herbal remedy, boiling smelly, stinky, lousy tasting bitter, sour herbs in a quart of water for three hours down to a pint. No effect. I then read **Ayurvedic Healing** by Dr. David Frawley, O.M.D. Ayurveda. My vegetarian diet: deficient protein, fat, excess cold, sweet (salads, fruit, juices, cold drinks, sugar) ⇨ eczema. I changed, ate more protein, fat (eggs, chicken, cheese, nuts, seeds), cooked vegetables, hot spices (7 per meal). Three weeks later: fully cured, no eczema just brand new, healthy, glowing skin and better digestion: less bloating, gas despite gaseous vegetables, beans. My friends were very happy.

Edema

Abnormal swelling, collection of fluids: within, between or under tissues, organs, skin, etc.

General causes:

1. Smoking, drugs, obesity, heart disease, diabetes

2. Cirrhosis, AIDS, infection, pregnancy, injury

3. Weak kidneys ⇨ edema: ankles, legs.
- Kidneys cleanse blood, remove water, minerals ⇨ urinary bladder ⇨ eliminated
- General causes: poor diet, excessive sex, diuretics, insomnia: CH. 10, 11, 16

4. Diet

a) Excess water via sugar, ice cream, salads, fruit, juices, smoothies, sodas, etc. ⇨ blood ⇨ body ⇨

- Arms, thighs ⇨ moist, white skin, pronounced swelling, holds imprint
- Lungs ⇨ excess water, mucus

b) Low protein (albumin) diet ⇨ extreme ⇨ disrupt fluid balance in the body ⇨
- Edema: dry skin, does not hold imprint

c) Excess protein ⇨ extreme ⇨ excess nitrogen in blood ⇨ kidneys ⇨ electrolyte, sodium, potassium imbalance ⇨
- Edema: swelling, redness, heat

Treatment: correct diet/ protein, diuretic foods, herbs
- Grains: corn, barley, rye, beans
- Celery, carrots, cranberries, asparagus
- Parsley, coriander, corn silk, lemon grass
- Avoid processed foods (generally high sodium)

General causes:
- Diet, excessive sex, diuretics, insomnia
- More info: CH. 10, 11, 16

d) Mineral imbalance.

Sodium (Na) via salt, food stimulates the kidneys, urination.
- Daily requirement: 2,300 mg (1 tsp. salt)
- Celery, medium stalk (30), steak 6 oz. (100)
- Processed foods, meals: high (read labels)

- Excessive sodium (>2300 mg. +/-) decreases potassium ⇨ edema

- Deficient sodium (<, +/-) ⇨ kidneys ⇨ excess renin (enzyme) ⇨ sodium retention ⇨ edema (arms, legs, heart, brain)

Potassium (K) via fruit, vegetables: natural diuretic, increases urination, eliminates sodium

Endometriosis

Abnormal growth of endometrial tissues (uterine mucus membrane lining) via too much protein, fat ⇨
- Premenstrual staining, nausea, vomiting
- Dysmenorrhea (painful menstruation)
- Painful urination, defecation, coitus
- Lower back pain, infertility

Treatment: CMD #2
- Bitters: turmeric, guggul, myrrh, dandelion
- +/- M.D.

Endometritis

Severe inflammation of endometrial tissue ⇨
- Infection, fever, vaginal discharge (foul)
- Enlargement of uterus
- Blockage in fallopian tube ⇨ ectopic pregnancy

General causes:

1. Bacterial infection (+/- sex)
2. Childbirth, IUD, abortion

3. Diet: excess protein, fat, sugar ⇨ blood ⇨ uterus

Treatment: CMD #2 (light diet)
- Spices: coriander, saffron, turmeric
- Aloe, dandelion, myrrh, golden seal, echinacea
- +/- M.D.

Fatigue

Exhaustion, weariness, loss of strength.

General causes
1. Diet: deficient protein, fat
2. Excess bitter herbs: laxatives, diuretics
3. Sex, excessive exercise, especially in A.M.

4. Coffee on empty stomach in A.M. ⇨ drop in blood sugar ⇨ fatigue
5. Sedentary lifestyle, pollution, smoking, drugs
6. Insomnia, heart, liver disease, diabetes, FMS

Fever

Rise in body temperature > normal (98.6°F) via
1. Stress, exercise, dehydration, obesity, climate
2. Infection (bacteria, viruses) ⇨ hypothalamus ⇨ raises T° ⇨ 103°F ⇨ burns, kills bacteria, viruses

Treatment:
- Bitter herbs (CH. 20, Cold, Flu)
- Rubbing the forehead, back of neck with ice
- Severe fevers: M.D.

Fibroid tumor (uterus)

Benign (harmless) fibrous tumor (fibroma) requires no surgery unless bleeding, discomfort.

General causes:
1. Obesity, genetics, estrogen supplements
2. Excess protein (animal, soy): increases estrogen

Treatment (dietary causes): CMD #1
- Kelp, spices, bitter herbs (golden seal)
- +/- M.D.

Fibromyalgia Syndrome (FMS)

Rheumatic (connective tissue) disorder

General symptoms: three months+

1. Chronic, achy, muscular, burning, throbbing, stabbing pain, stiffness, tender points ⇨ neck, shoulders, chest, back, thighs, especially in A.M.

2. Loss of balance, impaired coordination

3. Constipation, nauseas, gas, extreme fatigue

4. Anxiety, mood swings, nervousness, depression

5. Insomnia, dizziness, memory loss

6. Chemical or food allergies

7. Women: 30- 55

General causes:

1. Infections, poisons, injury, genetics

2. Weak digestion, IBS, Crohn's ⇨ excess poisons

3. Diet: low protein, fat, high raw vegetables, salads, juices, sugar, cold drinks

Treatment (dietary cause): HMD
- Ginseng, ashwagandha, turmeric
- +/- M.D.

Forgetfulness

Forgetfulness is temporary or permanent loss of memory. Blood (oxygen, protein, EFA, minerals, etc.) via arteries, capillaries build, fuel, moisten the brain (100 billion neurons).

General causes:

1. Anemia, deficient protein, fat, EFA; emaciation

2. Narrow, clogged coronary arteries, dry (smoking) or clogged lungs (water, mucus) reduce blood, oxygen ⇨ brain

3. Alcohol, drugs destroy brain cells; sex

TCM:

4. Deficient kidney yin (CH. 16) ⇨ short-term
   memory loss

5. Weak digestion decreases nutrient absorption,
   blood ⇨ brain ⇨ short-term memory loss

6. Heart (CH. 9): houses the mind ⇨ long-term
   memory

Treatment: middle diet, adjusted accordingly
- Smaller, simple meals
- Whole grains, almonds, sesame seeds, dairy
  help build brain tissue; gotu kola
- Reading, memory exercises, meditation, less sex

22. "G- H" DISEASES

Gallstones

Stones (calculus): gall bladder (cholelithiasis).

General causes:

1. Excess cholesterol, saturated fat, calcium salts
2. Insufficient bile salts, lecithin ⇨
- Crystallization of bile ⇨ pebble-like stones ⇨
- Congestion, obstruction of bile ⇨ GB, ducts ⇨
- Cholecystitis (GB inflammation) ⇨

General symptoms:
- Fever, nausea, vomiting, bitter taste (bile)
- Tea or coffee colored urine
- Pain: right side, upper abdomen (LV, GB) or behind breastbone: mimics heart attack
- Reversal of liver bile (yellow pigment) ⇨ blood ⇨ yellow skin, eyes (jaundice, CH. 23)

High fiber foods (whole grains, carrots, green beans, peas, tomatoes) help prevent formation of stones.

Three kinds:

1. Cholesterol (75%): animal, fried foods ⇨ yellow, green or red, sharp, pointy, painful gallstones

a) Treatment: mild pain
- CMD #1, turmeric, barberry (liver cleansing)
- Corn silk (1 oz./ 16 oz. water) + 2 tsp. coriander
- Lithotriptic (stone removing): dandelion, horsetail, parsley
- +/- M.D.

b) Treatment: severe: pain, fever
- Aloe vera, senna, rhubarb

- 3 TB olive oil, ½ lemon, juice in 2 C water before bed, two consecutive nights, sleep on right side, helps eliminate +/- pain
- +/- M.D.

2. Phlegm via dairy, cold drinks, sugar ⇨
- Round, soft, whitish, generally painless

Treatment: CMD #2
- Corn silk + coriander; parsley
- Dandelion, horsetail, turmeric, barberry
- +/- M.D.

3. Deficient protein, fat, cholesterol ⇨
- Black, brown, dry, rough, painful

Treatment: CMD #1 +/- chicken, turkey
- Corn silk tea, coriander, parsley
- +/- M.D.

GERD, GIRD

Gastro Esophageal Reflux Disease (GERD)
- Heartburn, burning pain: chest below sternum

Gastrointestinal Reflux Disorder (GIRD)
- Abdominal bloating, gas, nausea
- Acidic, sour taste in mouth, throat

General causes:

1. Diet
a) Deficient protein, fat, excess raw vegetables, fruit, juices, cold drinks weaken digestion ⇨
- Bloating, gas, nausea, acidity, malabsorption

Treatment: HMD, spices

Case history #32. Woman: dairy, beans, pasta, bread, salads, fruit, juices ⇨ bloating, gas, reflux, heartburn ⇨ medically diagnosed: **GIRD + menopause**.

I recommended HMD, fennel seeds (¼ tsp. after each meal). Three weeks later, she came back and hugged me. Her digestive problems and hot flashes had cured. I asked her age (43) and told her that clogged intestines had caused her hot flashes (why they disappeared) and not menopause, which I thought was an incorrect diagnosis. She was still menstruating regularly.

b) Excess fat, deficient fruit, vegetables ⇨
•   Food stagnation, reflux, acidity, heartburn, GERD

Treatment: CMD #1

c) Excess flour (pretzels, chips, etc.), oil ⇨ paste, narrow, clog stomach, pylorus (CH. 7) ⇨
•   Bloating, reflux, nausea (clogged pipe overflows)
•   Acidity, heartburn, GERD

Treatment: CMD #1
•   Vegetables (raw > cooked), mild spices, fruit
•   Smaller, earlier spaced meals

Case history #33. I (71), excess flour ⇨ narrow, clogged intestines ⇨ constant bloating, gas, reflux, nausea, pain, insomnia. I increased raw beets, carrots, celery, lettuce 2x/ day, no flour except toast (+ jelly). It took 3 weeks to cure. Age 72: history repeats itself, excess flour, ice cream (3 mos. ⇨ insomnia, 20# weight gain). Eight weeks to cleanse, lose 20#, sleep better.

d) Late dinners, snacks (after 6 P.M.), close meals, laying down after meals ⇨
•   Bloating, gas, acidity, malabsorption, insomnia

2. Pregnancy, tight clothing, belt, obesity

Gout

Type of arthritis via too much uric acid or defect in its metabolism ⇨ uric acid and its salts accumulate in the blood ⇨

- Joints: especially big toe ⇨
- Crystallize ⇨ needle shaped deposits ⇨
- Jabbing pain, inflammation
- Affects men (high animal) > women (low)

General causes:

1. Excess uric acid via diet

a) Red meat, beef, lamb, pork, venison, organ meats, seafood, shellfish, sardines, trout >> chicken, turkey high in **purines** >> peas, lentils, beans, etc. > oatmeal. Purines increase uric acid.
b) Alcohol, sugary foods, drinks

Treatment: CMD #1, 2
- Apples, grapes (¼ lb.), grapefruit, pumpkin, squash seeds help dissolve, eliminate uric acid
- Bitter herbs: sarsaparilla, guggul, yellow dock (blood cleansers), turmeric (digests protein)
- +/- M.D.

2. Deficient protein: decreases urinase (enzyme makes uric acid water-soluble)

Treatment: HMD (no red meat)
- Grapes, celery (raw)
- +/- M.D.

Hair

Hair is a living tissue that grows out of numerous follicles (sacs). It is nourished by jing, protein and fat (EFA). Most people lose 60 hairs/ day. After age 40, the number of hairs generally lessen and slowly lose color. Growth of hair after 70 slows. Baldness (alopecia) generally affects men more than women. General causes: heredity (grandparents), poor diet, drugs, excessive sex, hormonal imbalance, etc.

Jing/ ojas (sexual essence, ovum, sperm, etc.): fundamental substance of the body, hair, bones, etc.

- **Fountain of youth**: moist, firm skin, rich, colorful, thick hair, strong bones, etc. when full

- **Specter of old age**: gray, white, less hair, baldness, when in decline (varies)

Excessive sex, orgasm (daily, 3x/ week), worse when young or old (40+), coffee, caffeine, guarana, stimulants, insomnia consume excessively (CH. 16).

Long-term high protein, saturated fat, cholesterol ⇨ narrow coronary arteries, less blood to head ⇨ dry scalp, hair, skin loss, dandruff (white flakes).

Long-term low protein, fat, high raw vegetables, juices ⇨ anemia ⇨ hair loss, premature graying

Treatment: middle diet, adjusted accordingly
- Smaller meals: increases nutrient absorption
- Milk, ghee, amla, gotu kola
- Organic, ground black sesame seeds (unhulled), fenugreek seeds

- Saw palmetto, ashwagandha, zinc (supplement or pumpkin seeds, kelp), black pepper (increases nutrient absorption): 2x/ day for one month, may help rejuvenate hair follicles.

- Fo-Ti (gray hair, loss), sage

- Increase, darken hair: bhringraj (capsule, ground herb with food) and or scalp oil massage (+ hot water) 5 minutes (), let sit 5+ hours, then shampoo. Repeat 3x/ week.

- Reverse postures: slant boards, head stands increase blood flow to head

- Too many bitter herbs, coffee + low protein, fat dries the hair

Case history #13. 2013, I (vegan) added bitter herbs (cold, drying, extreme ⇨ poisonous) and coffee to my diet. A few months later, after a few beers ⇨ **red face**, **dizziness**, nausea, rapid heartbeat, **angina**, fever. I stopped the bitters, coffee, cured. Three days later, all my **hair** ⇨ **brittle**, **started breaking and falling out in clumps** ⇨ next three days starting from back ⇨ top ⇨ sides ⇨ front. I consulted a nurse, who looked under my eyes, at my nails and said I was anemic, iron deficient ⇨ hair loss. I started eating red meat, chicken (high iron), which immediately brought back heart symptoms. I stopped. I was not anemic just too little protein, fat and too much bitter, coffee ⇨ hair loss. I switched to CMD #1, dairy, sesame seeds, etc. My hair grew back.

Hay Fever (allergic rhinitis)

Chronic, respiratory allergy, seasonal via hypersensitive reaction to pollen, mold, dust ⇨
- Triggers immune response ⇨
- Itchy, watery eyes, runny, stuffed nose, sneezing

General causes:

1. Genetics: hypersensitive nervous system

2. Autoimmune disease

3. Constitution, diet

a) Vata or low protein, fat, excess cold, raw ⇨
- Dry lungs ⇨ hypersensitivity, coughing

Treatment: HMD (no red meat)
- Ginseng, astragalus, ashwagandha
- Avoid bitter herbs, coffee

b) Pitta or high protein, sugar ⇨ mucus, phlegm ⇨
• Lungs ⇨ clogged, hypersensitive, barking cough

Treatment: CMD #1
• Cilantro, bitters, echinacea
• Barberry, dandelion, burdock root

Coriander juice (a, b)

c) Kapha or cold, watery, sugar, dairy, fruit ⇨
• Blood ⇨ lungs ⇨ water, mucus, phlegm ⇨
• Clogged, hypersensitive
• Runny nose, watery eyes

Treatment: CMD #2
• Spices: dried ginger, basil + honey
• Clears mucus, phlegm, opens the sinuses

Headaches

General causes:

1. Muscular tension in head, neck, stress, worry

2. Dehydration, caffeine withdrawal, smoking, drugs

3. Sinusitis, allergies, sleep deprivation, eye strain

4. Electromagnetic radiation (computers, power lines)

5. High blood pressure, PMS, constipation, pollution

6. Constitution, body energies (Ayurveda, CH. 5)

a) Vata (air, wind) ⇨
• Throbbing, pulsing, fixed, irregular, migrating, sharp pain, headache (back of head)

General causes:
• Nervous exhaustion, excess worry, fear, anxiety

- Irregular routines, sleep, diet, missing meals
- Excess cold, dry, raw foods: caffeine, dehydration
- Excess stimulation (TV, computers)
- Indigestion, constipation, excess toxins in blood

b) Pitta (fire, bile, digestion) ⇨
- Sharp, intense, fever, burning pain ⇨ temples, behind eyes (red), center of head
- Oversensitivity to light, sound

General causes:
- Excess hot, spicy, fried, processed, sour (fermented), salty foods, drinks (alcohol, soy sauce, sauerkraut, etc.), caffeine, nicotine
- Stress, excess anger, frustration, sun, overwork
- Indigestion, hyperacidity, toxicity, etc.
- Liver (bile/ fat digestion) meridian ⇨ eyes

Treatment: CMD #1
- Aloe vera, gotu kola; sandalwood oil (forehead)
- Chamomile tea, honey

c) Kapha (water) ⇨
- Heavy, dull, throbbing pain ⇨ frontal headache
- Nausea, excess salivation, post-nasal drip

General cause: mucus congestion via
- Excessive: dairy, oily, cold, heavy foods
- Sedentary lifestyle, excessive sleep

Treatment: CMD #2
- Cloves, black pepper
- Ginger paste (forehead)

d) Coffee (acidic), caffeine (causes ST to overproduce acids) especially on empty stomach ⇨ overheats, irritates, burns the stomach ⇨
- Frontal headache

TCM: stomach meridian, energetic pathway passes through forehead ⇨ dull headache

Treatment: hot tea, soup

7. Migraine: vascular (blood vessel) headache via insomnia, stress, muscle tension, genetics ⇨
- Severe, intense, throbbing pain
- Nausea, oversensitivity (light, sound)
- Women (hormonal fluctuations) more than men

Treatment: good diet
- Chamomile, peppermint tea
- +/- M.D.

Hearing Loss

Sound ⇨ ears (3 parts)

1. Outer ear ⇨

2. Middle ear: eardrum canal, three tiny bones transmit, pass sound, vibrations ⇨

3. Inner ear: Corti, organ of hearing ⇨ auditory nerve ⇨ brain: heard, analyzed, defined

Hearing loss occurs when the passage of sound waves ⇨ brain ⇨ reduced or blocked.

Three kinds:

I. Conductive hearing loss: inadequate conduction of sound via external or middle ear

General causes:

A. External otitis (inflammation of outer ear) via cosmetics, piercing or bacterial infection

B. Changes in atmospheric pressure

C. Trauma, loud music, genetics

D. Bathing or swimming in contaminated water

E. Age 65+, clogged arteries, poor circulation, diabetes, obesity, anemia, infection, loud noise

F. Excess mucus, earwax, fluids in middle ear

Treatment:
- Ear candles place in ear, light the tip. As the cone, candle burns down, it absorbs water, wax, dries the ear. Stop when 2" from the ear. Ear candles, made with wax may drip into the ears.
- Hydrogen peroxide (1 TB) in ear (10 min.) helps dissolve, dislodge wax build up
- +/- M.D.

G. Diet

1. Excess soft dairy, juices, sugar, cold drinks, cold temperatures, winter, A/C ⇨
- Otitis media: inflammation, infection of middle ear via stagnant fluids ⇨ clog, pressurize ⇨
- Earache: sharp, dull or throbbing pain, high fever
- Common in infants, children: cold, watery

Treatment:
- Ear drops: garlic, echinacea, colloidal silver
- +/- M.D.

2. Excess building, saturated fat, oil, alcohol, liver congestion ⇨ tinnitus, loud ringing (CH. 26)

3. Deficient building ⇨ kidney yin deficiency (CH. 16) ⇨ tinnitus, low, soft ringing

II. Neural hearing loss via brain tumor or stroke

III. Sensorineural hearing loss, damage to auditory, inner ear nerves (acoustical) via virus's drugs, etc.

Internal otitis: inner ear inflamed via bacteria ⇨
- Hearing loss, vertigo, loss of balance, vomiting

Hearing deficit in infants, children:
- Inability to hear, especially high pitch sounds
- Failure to blink or react to loud noises
- Failure to turn head toward familiar sounds
- Mono-tonal babbling, shyness, withdrawal
- Failure to speak clearly by age two
- No interest in word games or being read to
- Habitual yelling, screaming when communicating
- Requires an M.D.

Heartburn

Backflow of HCL ⇨ esophagus via overeating ⇨
- Burning, stabbing pain in chest below sternum

Treatment:
- Raw lettuce, celery, water (dilutes, moves down)
- Red raspberry

Hemorrhoids (piles)

Bulging varicose veins around anus, above or outside anal sphincter ⇨ noticeable lumps, pain, itching, bleeding

General causes:
- Poor diet, laxatives, constipation
- Straining, squeezing, forcing evacuation
- Excessive sex, sedentary lifestyle, sitting

Three kinds (Ayurveda)

1. Dry, rough, painful via constipation, dry stools. old age, bed ridden

Treatment:
- Cooked, moist, oily foods, buttermilk; psyllium
- Sesame oil: rectum or enema (½ C) in evening

2. Swollen, red, painful +/- bleeding, pus via excess animal, sour, spicy, fried foods ⇨

Treatment: CMD #1
- Lotus root, pomegranate juice (external wash)
- Turmeric: internally, externally (paste)
- Avoid nightshades: potatoes, tomatoes, eggplant

3. Large slimy whitish, pale via dairy, eggs, sugar ⇨

Treatment: CMD #2
- Cayenne, black pepper, dried ginger, bayberry

Topical cures (I- III) twice daily
- 1 TB aloe vera gel plus little ginger
- Witch hazel, hammelis cream (homeopathic)

Hepatitis

Liver inflammation, viral infection via contaminated food, water, blood transfusions, needles, sex, etc.
- 25% ⇨ liver cirrhosis or cancer

General symptoms:
- Abdominal pain, fever, nausea, vomiting
- Dark urine, light-colored stools, loss of appetite
- Weakness, headaches, muscle aches, joint pain
- Drowsiness, jaundice (skin, eyes: yellow)
- Severe weight loss, death: hepatitis C

Treatment: CMD #1 (low fat), 2 + M.D.
- Bitters: aloe vera, golden seal, barberry, dandelion, gentian cleanses liver, purifies blood,
- Avoid alcohol, drugs, overeating

Herpes (genital)

Viral infection (toxin) via sexual contact ⇨ blood (toxic heat) ⇨ liver ⇨ overheats (liver heat) ⇨
- Liver meridian urinary, genital region ⇨
- Raised, red, painful skin eruptions, blisters
- Lesions, oozing sores that spread fast (wind, air)

Three kinds (Ayurveda):

1. Pitta, most common:
- Red, swollen, painful lesions, fever
- Worsened: animal, oily, fried, fermented foods, alcohol, wine, hot spices, overeating, smoking

Treatment: CMD #1
- Beets (raw), coriander, aloe vera, parsley
- Sarsaparilla, barberry, gentian, marshmallow
- Sores washed, douched w/ golden seal or gentian

2. Vata:
- Painful, hard lesions (not red or inflamed)
- Worsened by caffeine, low protein, fat

Treatment: CMD #1
- Milk, ghee, beets, ashwagandha, aloe vera
- Barberry, turmeric, sarsaparilla, gotu kola

3. Kapha:
- Weeping, oozing lesions (little redness, pain)
- Worsened by dairy, sugar, cold drinks

Treatment: CMD #2
- Spices: cayenne, dried ginger, cloves
- Bitters: aloe vera, barberry, turmeric, gentian

Case history #34. Woman (40's) customer, reduced her herpes (pitta) attacks to 1- 2 per year via vegetarian diet and herbs. Everything, including viruses lives and dies via favorite and non-favorite foods, herbs.

Acupuncture bleeds the eyes of the knees (dark capillaries on either side of patellar ligament, below knee cap) to lessen, cure.

High Blood Pressure

Blood pressure (BP): force of blood on arterial walls via <u>contraction</u> (<u>systolic</u>), expansion of the heart (CH. 9).

Normal BP: varies according to age, gender, etc.

1. Age 18- 39: female (<u>110</u>/68), male (<u>119</u>/70)
2. Age 40- 59: female (<u>122</u>/74, male (<u>124</u>/77)
3. Age 60+: female (<u>139</u>/68), male (<u>133</u>/68)
- Higher <u>systolic</u> # (varies) = high blood pressure
- Lower (90/60 varies) = low blood pressure
- Daytime (higher), night (lower)
- Stress, full bladder: higher

High blood pressure (hypertension) ⇨
- Palpitations, tachycardia, angina, insomnia
- Red face, irritability, heart attack, stroke, death

General causes:

1. Diet

a) Excess saturated fat, cholesterol (meat, chicken, turkey, eggs, dairy, butter) ⇨ clots, plaque ⇨ atherosclerosis ⇨ heart pumps faster ⇨ raises BP

b) Excess sodium (CH. 9) ⇨ kidneys ⇨ excess renin (enzyme) ⇨ sodium retention ⇨ edema ⇨ high BP

c) Inorganic calcium (white flour) ⇨ dries, hardens the arteries ⇨ arteriosclerosis ⇨ high BP

Treatment: CMD #1, 2
- Beets, lettuce, leafy greens (raw or juice), aloe

Case history #4. I (40- 70): HBP (150/110) via fatty, salty diet. I cured (weeks) each time via lacto-vegetarian/ vegan diet, vegetables, fruit, less eating, etc.

2. Age, smoking, vaping (CH. 8, 9) ⇨ dries arteries ⇨ arteriosclerosis ⇨ HBP (via insomnia, obesity)

3. Sex, stimulant drugs ⇨ adrenal glands ⇨ aldosterone (hormone) ⇨ sodium retention (1b)

High Cholesterol

General causes:

1. Liver disease (hepatitis, alcohol, etc.)

2. Diet: high saturated fat, cholesterol: meat, chicken, turkey, fish, butter, hard cheese, whole milk, palm coconut oil, fried foods, chocolate

Treatment: CMD #1, 2
- Fruit (apples, bananas, pears, strawberries, blueberries): pectin (high fiber)
- Carrots, beets, sweet potatoes, cauliflower, broccoli, spinach, kale, collard greens: high fiber reduces blood cholesterol, LDL, triglycerides
- Nuts, seeds, avocados olives, olive oil (EFA) ⇨ HDL ⇨ decrease LDL, cholesterol
- Spirulina, hawthorn berry, garlic
- More info: CH. 9 (Circulation)

Cholesterol lowering drugs, statins may cause fatigue, headaches, high blood sugar, diabetes. Eliminating high cholesterol foods is a better choice

Hot Flashes

Sudden feeling of warmth, temporary flushing, face, neck, chest, spike in body temperature, profuse perspiration, rapid heartbeat.

General causes:

1. Fluctuating or decreasing estrogen levels (menopause) ⇨ adversely affect hypothalamus (brain, regulates body temperature) ⇨ hot flashes

2. Stress, anxiety, certain medications, diseases

3. Constitution (Ayurveda, CH.5)

a) Vata (thin, dry, airy), low protein, fat diet ⇨
• Intermittent, periodic flashes

Treatment: HMD: dairy, chicken, turkey
• Aloe gel (reproductive organs), mild spices, sage
• Pear juice, peppermint tea, progesterone cream
• +/- M.D.

b) Pitta (hot, dry, oily)
• Excessive, frequent flashes

Treatment: CMD #1, 2, rest same as 2a.
• +/- M.D.

Case history #35. Progesterone cream, pear juice + peppermint tea. I (health food store, 17 yrs.) sold a lot and heard only praise.

Hyperacidity

Excess acid in small intestine (CH. 7) via

1. Overeating, poor food combining, meals too close
2. Excess spicy, sour foods, drinks: miso, soy sauce, pickles, sauerkraut, wine, alcohol, etc. ⇨
• Burping, acidic, sour taste, nausea, burning

Treatment:
• Water (+++), lettuce, celery; avoid juice
• Yogurt (unsweetened) +/- honey, etc.
• Aloe gel, licorice, gentian, barberry

Hyperglycemia

High blood sugar via excess sugar, concentrated, ice cream, candy, cookies, alcohol, etc.) ⇨
• Dry mouth, urine (sweet odor), hyperactivity
• More info: CH. 8 (Blood Sugar)

Treatment:
• Whole grains: sweet, reduce sugar cravings
• Golden seal, barberry, turmeric

Hyperkalemia

High blood potassium levels ⇨
- Nausea, diarrhea, muscle, heart weakness

General causes:
- Weak kidneys, excess diuretics
- Diet: high potassium (fruit, vegetables, beans, yogurt, etc.), low sodium (read labels)
- More info: CH 2 (Vitamins, Minerals, Enzymes), CH. 11 (Elimination)

Treatment: HMD
- More sodium: salt, animal
- +/- M.D

Hypoglycemia

Low blood sugar via

1. Excess insulin injection or secretion (via excessive sugar)

2. Drugs, glandular, kidney, pancreatic, liver, immune system disorders, diabetes mellitus

3. Diet: deficient protein, fat, sugar; fasting

General symptoms:
- Fatigue, headache, dizziness, sweating, nausea
- Palpitations, tremors, anxiety, confusion
- Swollen feet, constant hunger, craving for sweets
- Short temper, blurred vision, insomnia, coma

Treatment:
- Diet: carbohydrates (grain, sugar, etc.)
- +/- M. D.

Hypokalemia

Abnormally low blood levels of potassium ⇨
- Heart abnormalities

General causes:
- Adrenal tumor, starvation, diuretics
- Diet: excess sodium, deficient potassium

Treatment: more vegetables, fruit, less salt
- +/- M.D.

23. "I- O" DISEASES

Iatrogenic

Allopathy (drugs, surgery, etc.) while powerful and many times life-saving is an emergency medicine that kills disease to improve health, but many times harms. Johns Hopkins study (2019): **iatrogenic** (physician induced disease): 3rd leading cause of death (300,000). U.S.A. despite "best" doctors, medical care ranks:
- 26th out of 35 (world's democracies) in longevity
- 5th highest cancer, heart disease, diabetes, infant mortality rates
- Only 1 of 3 of 35 that allow pharmaceutical ads on television: deceptive, preys on fear.

Allopathy generally should not be the first treatment. Diet and herbs (generally safe, less harmful) is generally the first treatment if diet is the cause.

Impotence

Failure to achieve, maintain an erection or ejaculate. **Blood** (nutrients) via penile artery enlarges, elevates, hardens the penis. **Testosterone** ⇨ nerves ⇨ increases blood flow to penis ⇨ sexual desire, erection.

General causes:

1. Decline in testosterone via old age, excessive sex (CH. 16), chronic illness

2. Too little protein, fat, **cholesterol** ⇨ extreme ⇨ decrease testosterone (**steroid hormone**). Low fat or liver dysfunction ⇨ low cholesterol.

Treatment: HMD
- Meat, shellfish, eggs, dairy, sesame seeds, almonds, cashews increase jing, ojas (CH. 4, 5)

- Saw palmetto berry increases testosterone, potency, normalizes the prostate. Avoid if damp.
- Premature ejaculation: chestnut, lotus seed, nutmeg
- Pumpkin seeds (prostate), Solomon's Seal
- No sex, etc. until stronger
- +/- M.D.

Case history #16. I (20- 26) premature ejaculation, impotence via vegetarian diet, worse the more vegan, raw I ate. I cured with meat, chicken, turkey.

Case history #17 (store). Man (30's): impotent last four months: new girlfriend (vegan). He had stopped eating meat, chicken, etc. became weak, impotent. I advised dairy, eggs and make a gradual transition +/-.

3. Excess protein, sat. fat, cholesterol ⇨ extreme ⇨
- Clogs, narrows penile artery ⇨ less blood to penis

Treatment: CMD #1, 2
- Pumpkin seeds, saw palmetto

Infertility

Inability to conceive: function of ovum, sperm, hormones, blood, diet, age, genetics, etc.

General causes:

1. Ovulation disorders via:
a) Fibroids, pelvic inflammatory disease
b) Polycystic ovary syndrome, endometriosis
c) Uterus (abnormal), blocked fallopian tubes

2. Man (low sperm count) via excessive sex, low protein, fat diet, age, etc. More info: CH. 16

3. Diet

a) Deficient protein, fat (animal > plant) ⇨ extreme ⇨ less estrogen, blood ⇨ infertility, miscarriage

Treatment: HMD
- Red meat, chicken, turkey, dairy, sesame seeds
- Cooked vegetables (roots, round), royal jelly
- Saw palmetto berry: underdeveloped breasts, ovaries; ashwagandha, Solomon's seal, saffron
- Siberian ginseng (digestion), nettles (estrogen)
- Evening primrose, black currant oil, marshmallow
- Less sex, avoid bitter herbs, coffee
- +/- M.D.

Case history #6. Woman (mid 30's), macrobiotic diet (vegan, low protein, fat) ⇨ deficiency ⇨ lack of holding ⇨ four miscarriages. I recommended HMD, red meat, chicken or turkey 2x daily, cooked vegetables, Evening Primrose Oil, Siberian ginseng to build blood, strengthen sex organs, wait 4 months (new blood) before trying to get pregnant. She now has two healthy boys.

4. Excess saturated fat, cholesterol, trans fats thicken congest sex organs ⇨ #1a- c, infertility

Treatment: CMD #1, 2
- Myrrh: moves blood, cleanses uterus
- + M.D.

Inflammation

Natural response: swelling, burning pain, redness of bodily tissues, fever, loss of function, etc.

General causes:

1. Dryness, injury, poisons, infection, bacteria, virus

2. Diet

a) Excess fat, cholesterol ⇨ narrow, clogged arteries ⇨ reduced circulation, blood (moistening) ⇨ arms, legs, muscles, tendons, etc. (moist: smooth, easy movement, expansion, contraction) ⇨
- Dry ⇨ inflammation, pain, arthritis (CH. 19)

Treatment: CMD #1 (anti-inflammatory)
- Dairy, vegetables, fruit, nuts, seeds (EFA)
- Bitters (anti-inflammatory): turmeric, wild cherry bark, white willow bark, mullein (nerve); spirulina

3. Deficient protein, fat (builds, fuels moistens) ⇨ dryness, inflammation, loss of function

4. Alcohol, caffeine, processed foods, smoking

Case history #36. I (49) driving with my elbow bent, hanging out the window. Six hours later became numb and so painful that I considered going to a hospital but instead went to my hotel. I realized the pain was due to bent elbow ⇨ decreased blood flow ⇨ inflammation. I put camphor oil (White flour), very hot, wrapped with plastic to trap, concentrate the heat ⇨ elbow ⇨ improved circulation, blood flow. An hour later, my arm felt cold, sweaty. I removed the plastic, dried my arm. No pain.

Insomnia

Sleeping rejuvenates the body mind via connection with one's spirit (Spirit) and not food, water or air. Normal, deep sleep: 6- 8 hours +/- ⇨
- Better, easier in youth (more jing, health)
- Worse, harder, shorter in old age (less jing)
- Need to sleep long hours declines with age
- Best times: 10 P.M. – 6 A.M., atmosphere negatively charged

Insomnia: difficulty or inability to fall or stay asleep, shallow, dream disturbed or unsatisfying sleep.
- Two types:

I. Acute (sudden onset)

General causes:
- Nervousness, worry, anxiety, stimulant drugs
- Caffeine (lasts 11 hours), late meals, overeating
- Excess spicy, sour foods, drinks, change in diet

- Excess nighttime stimulation: reading, TV, etc.

II. Chronic

General causes:

1. Diet

a) Deficient protein, fat, excess bitters, coffee ⇨
- Inability to fall asleep, easily disturbed
- Frightening dreams, nightmares, flying
- Wakes up often, difficulty falling back to sleep

Treatment: HMD
- Sweet, heavy, grounding, moistening foods
- Turkey, eggs, dairy (milk)
- **Walnuts** (¼C): **melatonin** (hormone regulates sleep cycle, decreases with age), **tryptophan** (amino acid produces melatonin, **serotonin**: **neurotransmitters**: regulate mood, sleep cycle), **magnesium** (relaxes muscles, nervous system, easier to fall, stay asleep), **potassium**, **calcium** (sleep), omega–6 fatty acids
- Whole grains (complex sugar) stabilize blood sugar levels, prevent nighttime spikes or drops ⇨ awakening. Oats (melatonin, magnesium)
- Cooked carrots, hard squash, potatoes, yams
- **Raisins**: melatonin, sugar (releases slowly into blood stream, stabilizes blood sugar), fiber (improves digestion, nighttime indigestion: awakening)
- Nutmeg (in warm milk) or valerian before bed

Case history #37. I (69), vegan, dry, low protein, fat, bitter herbs, coffee ⇨ angina (chest, left arm pain) ⇨ severe insomnia. I stopped the beans, bitters, etc. increased cooked vegetables, fruit, eggs and milk. The angina disappeared and I slept better: quicker, deeper.

Case history #38. I (72), lacto-vegetarian started eating less cheese and more raw vegetables (3+), 2x/day ⇨ severe insomnia, could not fall or stay asleep.

My BP dropped ⇨ 110/ 70: good. My resting heartbeat dropped ⇨ low 50's, high 40's (not good): heart weakness. This lasted four weeks until I figured it out, increased yogurt, cheese, cooked vegetables ⇨ normal heartbeat.

b) Excess building, animal, fat, cholesterol ⇨
- Clogged arteries, hypertension, obesity, slow digestion, peristalsis (downward movement of food, stools), clogged intestines ⇨
- Increases energy, heat, fire, body temperature ⇨
- Difficulty falling or staying asleep (11 P.M. ⇨ 3 A.M.)

Treatment: CMD #1, 2
- Walnuts, 50% vegetables (raw > cooked), fruit
- Green vegetable juices, raisins; milk thistle
- Valerian, skullcap (vasodilator), gotu kola
- Niacin: 50 mg. (lessens or eliminates body flush, skin irritation: 20 minutes.

Case history #39. I (40's): clogged arteries, high blood pressure via overeating, red meat, chicken, etc. ⇨ horrific insomnia, could not fall or stay asleep, until 5:00 A.M. ⇨ short sleep (2 hrs.). I changed my diet: CMD #1: 2 months ⇨ 15 lb. weight loss, lower BP, better sleep.

c) Excess water, protein, sugar (sugar, honey, dairy, fruit, beer, etc.) ⇨ blood ⇨ lungs ⇨
- Excess water, mucus ⇨ obstructs, stops breath during sleep ⇨ gasping, wakefulness, sleep apnea

Treatment: CMD #2
- Barley, quinoa, azuki beans, walnuts
- Spices: cardamom, garlic, ginger
- Nose strips contain spices (essential oils): open, the nose, sinuses expand, ventilate the lungs

Case history #22. I (71, lacto-vegetarian), ice cream, vegie burgers, chocolate (high fat) ⇨ 2 weeks ⇨ severe chest pain ⇨ insomnia. I stopped the ice cream, etc., took one week to cure. I went from extreme (low fat) to the other (high fat) ⇨ clogged coronary arteries.

d) Excess flour (bread, noodles, cookies, pretzels, chips) ⇨ extreme (weeks, months) ⇨ pastes, clogs small intestine (SI) ⇨
- Bloating, gas, pain, acidity, reflux, nausea ⇨
- Frequent awakenings, difficulty returning to sleep

Treatment:
- More raw vegetables, fruit, juices, raisins
- Water (3+ glasses/ day), less or no flour

Case history #40. I (71) cookies, chips, clogged SI ⇨ constant bloating, gas, reflux, nausea, pain ⇨ severe insomnia. I changed my diet, more raw vegetables (3+, 2x/day), less flour, except toast (+ jelly). It took three weeks to cure. Age 72: history repeats, flour + ice cream (3 months, 20# weight gain): 8 weeks to cure, eliminate.

2. Hypoglycemia (low blood sugar) ⇨ night ⇨
- Restlessness ⇨ wakefulness, fragmented sleep ⇨
- Wake up tired, feeling heavy

General dietary causes: deficient protein, fat; fasting

Treatment: #1a +/- M.D.
- More info: CH. 8, 21, 22

3. Obesity insulates, overheats the body

4. Arthritis, diabetes, drugs, chronic illness

5. Physical, mental tension

Treatment:
- Yoga before or in bed: corpse position (lying flat on back), head/ pillow, alternately tensing, relaxing body ⇨ feet, ankles, legs, abdomen, chest, arms, hands, neck, shoulders ⇨ head
- Deep abdominal breathing, especially left nostril
- Sleeping on **right side** opens **left** nostril (cools, relaxes); **left** side opens **right** nostril (heats)
- Sound sleep occurs via either nostril
- Avoid sleeping face-down on stomach

The thoughts you have before falling asleep can be the thoughts you wake up with. Think positive.

Irritable Bowel Syndrome (IBS)

IBS (intestinal neurosis, spastic colitis): chronic digestive, eliminative disorder ⇨
- Abdominal cramping, nausea, excessive gas
- Constipation, diarrhea, inability to empty bowels
- Anxiety, depression, loss of appetite
- Attacks women (weak digestion via menstruation, cold, low protein, fat diet) > men (testosterone, high protein, fat, strong digestion)

General causes:

1. Low protein, fat, excess dairy, sugar, cold, drinks, salads, fruit, juices, smoothies, sodas, etc. cool, dilute, weaken, slow, stop digestion, elimination

Treatment: CMD #2
- Cooked > raw vegetables, black pepper

Case history #10. Woman (35, S. FL): **IBS**: bloating, gas, nausea, loose stools, swollen arms (3x normal) via cold, sweet low protein, fat dairy, pasta, salads, fruit, sugar, juices, sodas, etc. I recommended cooked vegetables, spices (5+), beans +/- chicken, no dairy. **Nine** months later, all symptoms gone. She was very happy but still worried, saw a nutritionist ($300): stool sample (high bacteria), sold her **golden seal** (bitter, cold, antibacterial), 9 caps/ day. Three weeks came to my store to buy more. I asked why, who, how long, results? All her gastro-intestinal symptoms had returned. I explained. **Bitter herbs** (except turmeric) kill bacteria including healthy digestive bacteria. 9 caps/ day (extreme) was appropriate for edema, infections or inflammation (which she did not have), but not someone cold, deficient, still recovering, which is why she reacted so poorly, quickly. I refused the sale, had her continue original diet, spices, etc. She recovered.

2. Gastro-intestinal infections, antibiotics
3. Mental trauma, stress, allergies, etc.

Jaundice

Yellowing of skin or eyes (whites) via abnormal accumulation of bilirubin (yellow pigment: bile) in blood.

General causes:

1. Diet: excess saturated fat, cholesterol ⇨ gallstones (CH. 22) ⇨ obstruct gall bladder, ducts ⇨ reversal of bile flow ⇨ liver ⇨ blood ⇨ skin, eyes

Treatment: CMD #1, 2
- Mild spices, raw, cooked vegetables
- Dandelion, barberry, aloe, no alcohol
- + M.D.

2. Liver disease, tumors, parasites
3. Pernicious anemia (vitamin B-12 deficiency)
4. Death of red blood cells (120-day life-span)
5. Common in newborn babies

Kidney Stones

Excess minerals or uric acid via diet or malfunctioning parathyroid gland ⇨ stones (renal urinary calculus) ⇨ kidneys, ureter, urinary bladder ⇨
- Frequent urination (odorous, cloudy +/- pus, blood)
- Chills, fever, profuse sweating
- Pain radiating from groin, abdomen to upper back
- Urinary tract infection, dysuria (+ blood)
- Affects mostly white men 30-50: high protein, fat

Four kinds:

1. Calcium oxalate (#1: 80%) via excess
- Fish, eggs, dairy, asparagus, tomatoes, potatoes
- Eggplant, spinach, beets, rhubarb, blueberries

2. Struvite (infection stones) more so in women: UTI

3. Uric acid (red, yellow, painful): extremely high levels via excess protein or deficient urination

4. Cystine (congenital defect)

Treatment: CMD 2
- Distilled water (thins urine, stones), radishes
- Diuretics: cranberry juice; corn silk, parsley, uva ursi, juniper berry, sarsaparilla, coriander, fennel ⇨ increase urination, help eliminate stones
- Lithotriptic herbs dissolve stones, short-term use: horsetail (irritant), burdock root, yellow dock
- Pumpkin, squash seeds (tea)
- Avoid enriched flour, calcium supplements
- Panful to eliminate
- +/- M.D.

Laryngitis

Dryness or inflammation of mucus membrane lining of larynx (vocal cords) ⇨ loss or hoarseness of voice.

General causes:

1. Diet

a) Excess dairy, sugar, fruit, juices, cold drinks ⇨
- Phlegm ⇨ pastes, obstructs throat, larynx

Treatment: CMD #2, cloves, barberry, golden seal

b) Low protein, fat, high raw fruit, vegetables ⇨
- Dry throat, larynx ⇨ laryngitis

Treatment: HMD (no red meat) or CMD #1
- Marshmallow, licorice tea, slippery elm lozenges

c) High protein, fat (animal), fried foods, sugar ⇨
- Yellow mucus, severe sore throat ⇨ laryngitis

Treatment: CMD #1
- Turmeric, barberry

2. Viruses, excessive talking, smoking, etc.

Low Blood Pressure

Low blood pressure (hypotension): 90/60 (+/-) ⇨
- Palpitations, poor memory, dizziness, anxiety
- Insomnia, dream-disturbed sleep, pale lips
- Blurred vision, fatigue, dull-pale complexion

General causes:
1. Anemia, debility, malnutrition, hemorrhage
2. Dehydration (blood: 92% water), medications
3. Heart, liver, kidney disease
4. Overactive vagus nerve,
5. High blood pressure (CH. 22) ⇨ extreme ⇨ weakens heart ⇨ low BP

6. Diet:

a) Long-term low protein, fat, high fruit, vegetables ⇨ weaken heart, slow pumping ⇨ lowers BP

Treatment (CH. 9): HMD (no red meat)
- Dairy, eggs, vegetables (cooked > raw)
- Spices: cinnamon, ginger, cayenne, garlic

b) Excess dairy, salads, juices, sugar, etc. ⇨
- Mucus, phlegm congestion in lungs ⇨ reduces oxygen ⇨ hypoxemia, stresses, weakens heart

Treatment: CMD #2, spices

Malabsorption

Little or no nutrient absorption (SI, LI) ⇨
- Loss of appetite, bloating, weight loss, fatigue
- Loose stools (high fat content), muscle pain
- Fingernails: poor formation, spots, ridges

General causes:

1. Drugs, bacterial infections

2. Chronic illness, cystic fibrosis, celiac disease

3. Diet

a) Excess fat, oil, flour ⇨ pastes, clogs SI, LI ⇨
• Reduces digestion, nutrient absorption

Treatment: CMD #1
• Coriander, fennel, turmeric, ashwagandha

b) Deficient protein, fat
c) Excess fruit, juices, sodas, cold drinks, fluids with
   or after meals, raw vegetables
d) Irregular diet, eating habits (CH. 7) ⇨
• Weak digestion, poor nutrient absorption
• Greater waste, poisons

Treatment: HMD (no red meat)
• Whole grains, basmati rice, potatoes
• Spices: ginger, cardamom, nutmeg
• Saw palmetto, ashwagandha

Treatment: CMD #2

Menorrhagia, metrorrhagia

Menorrhagia: abnormally long, heavy menses or spotting between. Metrorrhagia: uterine bleeding.

General causes:

1. Smoking, alcohol, birth control pills, abortion

2. IUD, endometritis, polyp, tumor, cervical cancer

3. Diet: overeating, hot, spicy, sour, oily, salty foods

Treatment: CMD #1
- Red raspberry leaf, yarrow, milk thistle (1)
- Aloe, ashwagandha, Bhringraj, amalaki
- +/- M.D.

Miscarriage

General causes:

1. Spiritual. It is not meant to be, has nothing to do with mother or father.
2. Diet: too little protein, fat, too much coffee

Case history #6. 1997 Woman (36): macrobiotic diet, mostly vegan (low protein, fat), salads, juices, some cheese ⇨ anemia, deficiency, lack of holding ⇨ 4 **miscarriages**. I recommended: red meat, chicken or turkey 2x/day, cooked vegetables, Siberian ginseng, Evening Primrose Oil to build blood, strengthen sex organs, and waiting **4** months (new, greater protein, fat, blood) before trying. She now has two healthy boys.

Multiple Sclerosis

Progressive nervous system disorder disease via deterioration of myelin sheath (white fatty substance covers some nerve fibers): diagnosed via MRI or spinal tap.

General symptoms:
- Malfunctioning nerves, immune system
- Dizziness, fatigue, blurred or double vision
- Stiff muscles, tingling, numbness (hands, feet)
- Loss of balance, falling, impaired speech
- Women (25- 40): menstruation, low protein, fat diet > men (high protein, fat)

General causes:
- Poisons, pesticides, mercury, drugs
- Genetics, radiation
- Diet: processed foods, fat, sugar, chemicals

Misdiagnosis, mistreatment can occur without verification (MRI, spinal tap) as MS shares similar symptoms (fatigue, dizziness, stiffness, numbness, etc.) with low protein, fat diet, anemia, atherosclerosis. More info: CH. 24 (Pharmaceutical Drugs, case history).

Nails

Nails: largely keratin (protein), minerals via diet. It takes seven months to grow: bottom (base) to top (end).

General symptoms:
- Round, curved or spoon shaped
- Thin, dry, brittle, cracked, hangnails
- Horizontal or vertical ridges, white spots, fungus

General causes:
1. Deficient protein, fat: brittle, cracked
2. Deficient iron: spoon shaped
3. Deficient calcium, zinc, excess sugar: white spots

Treatment: HMD, CMD #1
- Sesame seeds (unhulled, black > brown), flaxseed, almonds, walnuts, high protein, EFA, minerals
- Amla, silica (minerals)

Case history #42. I (63, vegetarian): cracked nails (pinkie, thumb), cured quickly: sesame seeds, walnuts.

4. Fungus, worms, parasites ⇨ ridges, cracks
- General causes: diet, hot, damp, tropical climate

Treatment (+ M.D.):
- Bitter herbs (internal): CH 26 (worms)
- Topical: Australian tea tree oil or vinegar and water rinse

Nausea

Urge to vomit. General causes:

1. Overeating, pregnancy, obesity, tight belts ⇨ obstruct ST, SI (CH. 7, Digestion), downward movement of food ⇨ collects ⇨ backs up ⇨ overflows ⇨ nausea

2. Impure foods, bacteria, viruses, motion sickness

Treatment: acute (sudden)
- Water, raspberry leaf tea: avoid if thin, dry, tight
- Ginger: food stagnation, motion sickness
- +/- M.D.

Treatment:
- More vegetables (raw > cooked), fruit, juice
- More info: CH. 7 (Digestion), 22 (GIRD)

Neuralgia

Severe, burning pain along the course of nerve. Blood, nutrients (protein, fat) build, moisten the nerves.

General causes:

1. Nerve damage, trauma, diabetes, shingles

2. Lyme disease, syphilis

3. Diet: too little protein, fat ⇨ extreme ⇨ weakens, thins, dries, inflames, pains nerves, muscles, etc.

Case history #9. Woman (26, athlete), **neuralgia**: severe foot pain, trouble walking, standing, wheelchair (airport), seen doctors, orthopedic surgeons, blood work, x-rays, MRI, acupuncturists, chiropractors, to no avail. I diagnosed blood deficiency, anemia via long-term low protein, fat diet, starting early (teens) ⇨ less blood, jing ⇨ legs, muscles, nerves, etc. ⇨ dried, inflamed, severe pain. I recommended: HMD, red meat every day. A year later, 80% better, able to walk, stand and exercise without pain or fear, cured fully when she decided to eat red meat 2x/ day.

Numbness

Partial or total lack of sensation in the body. Blood (nutrients, protein, fat, etc.) via capillaries, arteries, etc. stimulate, build, fuel, moisten the nerves, muscles, etc.

General causes:

1. Injury, nerve damage, anemia

2. Decreased circulation, blood via winter, sedentary lifestyle

3. Diet

a) Too little protein, fat dries, weakens, pains

b) Too much protein, fat ⇨ narrow arteries (chest) ⇨ reduces circulation, blood ⇨ arms, legs

Treatment middle diet adjusted accordingly
*   Exercise, weight loss if necessary
*   Massage, hot compresses
*   +/- M.D.

Case history #36. I (49) driving to Colorado with my elbow, bent hanging out the open window. Six hours later, my elbow became numb and so painful that I considered going to a hospital, but instead went to a hotel, where I figured out, realized that the pain was due to the bent elbow: decreased circulation ⇨ dryness, inflammation, pain. I put camphor oil (White flour): very hot, wrapped with plastic (trap, concentrate heat) ⇨ improve circulation, blood ⇨ elbow. An hour later, my arm felt cold, sweaty. I removed the plastic, dried my arm. No pain.

Obesity

Excess body weight (protein, fat, flour, water): 20% greater than normal ⇨

- Heart disease, insomnia, arthritis

- Weak immunity

- Diabetes (CH. 21) via insulin resistance

General causes:

1. Diet: overeating
a) Meat, fish, eggs, dairy, oil, bread, cookies, chips
b) Excess sugar (natural, synthetic, fruit, juice, alcohol, etc.) ⇨ fat ⇨ skin (insulation, energy)

Treatment: CMD #1, 2, two meals/ day
- Whole grains, cooked, raw vegetables
- Mild spices: cumin, coriander, fennel, turmeric
- Bitters: aloe, barberry, turmeric, milk thistle

2. Constitution: kapha (CH.5, Ayurveda)

3. Sedentary lifestyle, hypothyroid, high stress

4. Certain diseases, medications, advertising

A wise person controls the future, loses weight by controlling the present, refrigerator:
- Stock more yogurt, nuts, seeds, vegetables, fruits, juices, bread, sugar free jelly, honey, etc.
- Less junk (cookies, ice cream, chips, beer, soda)

You cannot eat what is not there, but instead will be forced to eat what is there, and eventually will not miss what is not there. Habits are easy to make and break. Bad habits can be replaced with good habits. The more natural, healthier you eat, the greater distaste for junk, high fat, sugar, old, artificial, poisonous foods, drinks.

The more junk you stock, the MORE you eat, weigh, suffer. Is today's **10 minutes** of junk, pleasure **worth** tomorrow's disease, dental decay, extra weight and a longer, more restrictive, corrective diet, herbs?

If you must eat junk buy **small** amounts. You do not have to eat the worst sweet. **Sweet is sweet**. Fruit, toast, jelly, yogurt + honey (ice cream substitute) while not cookies, ice cream, etc. is still sweet, fills up the stomach ⇨ reduces hunger, appetite, sweet cravings.

Everything is a choice. Resolve to be different, better, more disciplined, one meal, day at a time. Have patience when older as it is easy, fast, days to put on weight, longer, weeks to lose.

Case history #43. I used to give a woman (37) and her children a ride whenever I saw them walking. One time, we talked about health and I gave her a copy of my book. I saw her two months later. She had read my book, changed her diet, lost 17#.

Case history #44. I (60): 20 lbs. overweight needed to lose weight to fit into a 20-year-old suit for my niece's wedding. Lost 20# in 4 months via CMD, salads, fruit juices (with pulp), less grain and walking.

Osteoporosis

Bone loss is natural with age: Abnormal loss of bone tissue ⇨ thin, brittle bones, fracture ⇨ women (age 50+) > men (65+). Jing (CH. 16), protein, fat: substances, glue: holds minerals, solidifies bones.

General causes:

1. Low jing via excess sex, childbirth, long-term: low protein, fat diet

2. Gender: women smaller, thinner, less dense bones, menopause (CH. 16), decline in estrogen suffer osteoporosis 80% >men

3. Diet: meat, chicken, turkey, caffeine, sugar ⇨ acidic, leaches calcium: bones, teeth

Treatment: middle diet, adjusted accordingly
- Seeds: raw, ground sesame, flax: high EFA
- Leafy greens, fish oil (EFA)
- More info: CH 20 (Bones)
- +/- M.D.

4. Diuretics (water pills) increase calcium excretion
   ⇨ extreme (years) ⇨ fractures

5. Sedentary lifestyle weakens

6. Endocrine disorder, steroids

24. "P" DISEASES

Pancreatitis

Inflammation of pancreas (behind stomach, lower left-side ribcage) ⇨
- Upper abdominal swelling, nausea, vomiting
- Severe, burning, stabbing pain around navel, radiates to back

General causes:

1. Alcoholism, hepatitis

2. Diet: high fat, triglycerides, sugar, animal

Treatment: CMD #1, 2
- Vegetables (raw> cooked), mild spices
- Bitter herbs, roots (golden seal, gentian, burdock, dandelion) increase bile ⇨ reduces digestive strain on pancreas, as does lesser fat, animal, etc.
- +/- M.D.

Pediatric Illnesses

Children: dominated by water, still developing, weak fire ⇨ weak, watery digestion, immunity, respiration ⇨
- Bloating, gas, reflux, pain, malabsorption
- Colds, flus, sore throat, swollen glands
- Mucus, bacteria, viruses, ear infections, etc.

Best foods (after breast milk) for growth, development:
- Organically grown nuts, seeds (raw, ground), grains (whole > flour)
- Fresh fruit, vegetables, juices, water (room T°)
- Dairy (hormone, antibiotic free), sesame oil
- Animal flesh: difficult to digest, cleanse
- +/- M.D.

Protein, fat build, fuel all structure function.

1. **Milk**: cow (mucus forming)
a) Best digested alone, boiled w/ spices: cardamom, ginger, cinnamon: reduce mucus; or with whole grains (rice), sweet fruit (bananas, papayas)
b) Poor combinations ⇨ gas, acidity
• Sour fruit, meat (red, white), fish
• Milk, cereal (flour, sugar)
c) Non-dairy (soy, rice): lesser mucus, fat
d) Ice cream (all): cold, high fat, sugar, mucus

Raw milk: like breast milk: alive, easily absorbable protein, vitamins, minerals, enzymes (lactase), probiotics (digestive bacteria). U.S. (9 million users, 17 states legal. Number: sicknesses, deaths: extremely low.

Pasteurization (ultra-heating) kills most vitamins, enzymes, bacteria (including beneficial), which is why pasteurized milk is fortified. Ask M.D.

2. **Yogurt**: calcium, potassium, magnesium, probiotics, mucus, digests well with vegetables, spices (cardamom, coriander, cumin); poorly with milk, nuts, sour fruit. Best bought unsweetened. Add honey, maple syrup or fruit to sweeten.

3. **Cheese**: most mucus forming (Swiss: least) does not combine well with animal, grain, beans, nuts, seeds. Mustard, cumin, cardamom helps digest.

4. **Nuts** (almonds, walnuts), **seeds** (sesame, flax), raw, unhulled, ground: high protein, EFA: bones, teeth, hair

5. **Whole grains** (rice, barley, millet, buckwheat, rye). Flour (pretzels, chips, cookies, etc.): less nutrition, pastes intestines: bloating, reflux, malabsorption

Water, minerals, enzymes, fiber cleanse, purify, etc.

6. **Vegetables**: cooked > raw. Cooked potatoes, hard squash, carrots, roots, sweet vegetables, fiber improve digestion, elimination. Dessert (sugar substitute): cooked sweet potatoes, hard squash, pumpkin, raw carrots + ginger, cinnamon

Vegetables (vital to health, cleanses poisons, waste) are generally the biggest stumbling block. 17 years (health food store): talked to many women, some whose children (indigestion, constipation, colds, flus) ate few vegetables. I asked why? "My child does not like vegetables." I told them their children would suffer more sicknesses unless they became stricter and more creative, better recipes, sweet vegetables, spices, etc. As a child I had to eat all my vegetables before I could eat dessert or leave the table. Fortunately, I liked most vegetables. I also eventually took cooking classes, which helped me make tasty, healthy meals, which is exactly what parents must do to get their kids to eat vegetables. which is why this book has a cooking class. Parenting is a spiritual dictatorship. Do what it takes.

7. **Fruit**: raw, cooked (+ raisins, cinnamon, ginger, cardamom: immunity), juice (unsweetened)

8. **Sugar** (natural): honey, maple syrup, sugar cane

9. **Spices** (mild, hot, dry): ginger, cardamom, cinnamon, coriander, fennel, cumin
- Increase digestion, reduce mucus, phlegm
- Improve immunity, kill bacteria, viruses
- Best consumed, small amounts with dairy, grain, vegetables, soup, desserts. Avoid peppers.

PATHOLOGIES (age 3+)

1. Deficient protein, fat (animal, plant) ⇨
- Anemia, weak function, colds, flus

2. Too little EFA ⇨ poor mental development, learning disorders

3. Excess protein, fat (animal, plant), oil, sugar ⇨
• Bloating, pain, acidity, heartburn, obesity

4. Excess beans, flour, raw vegetables ⇨
• Abdominal bloating, gas, pain
• Malabsorption, constipation

5. Deficient cleansing, vegetables
• Bloating, pain, hard abdomen, constipation

6. Excess cold drinks, ice water, juice, soda, etc. ⇨
• Bloating, gas, malabsorption, loose stools

Treatment: diet + M.D.

7. Excess protein, sugar via dairy, fruit, desserts, etc. ⇨ blood ⇨ lungs ⇨ excess water, mucus ⇨
• Coughing, sneezing, cold, flu (virus)
• Bacteria, viruses thrive in stagnant fluids

Treatment: CMD #2
• Whole grains, nuts, seeds, spices
• Cooked vegetables with ghee or sesame oil
• +/- M.D.

8. Middle ear infection
• Fever, earache (sharp or dull, throbbing pain)

Treatment:
• Garlic or peppermint oil (1-2 drops, mix with 1 tsp. water) ⇨ ear ⇨ dries, destroys infection
• Older children: ear cones (wax, non-wax). Place in ear, light exposed end. As cone burns down, wax is drawn up, out. Pull out (1½" left) before burning ear. Wax candles may drip wax into ears.
• +/- M.D.

9. Hearing deficit (infants, children):
• Inability to hear, especially high pitch sounds
• Failure to blink or react to loud noises
• More info: CH. 22 (Hearing Loss)

Control what your child eats. Do not stock junk. Eat the same diet, foods if you want your children to follow your good and not theoretical example. The good, natural foods you eat will eventually take over, increase taste, desire for healthy foods and distaste for junk, especially when not feeling well. Talk about sugar, tooth decay, root canals, etc. Show your teeth, new, repaired.

Avoid **vaccines** preserved with **mercury** ⇨ **autism**.

Pelvic Inflammatory Disease

General symptoms:
- Fatigue, fever, chills, vaginal discharge (foul)
- Pain: pelvis, abdomen, lower back, vagina, during sexual intercourse or urination

General causes:

1. Bacterial infection via sex, chlamydia, gonorrhea
2. Vaginal infection, childbirth, miscarriage

3. Excess fat, oil, spicy sour foods, drinks, sugar ⇨

Treatment: CMD #2
- Myrrh, turmeric, coriander, saffron
- Aloe vera gel, sarsaparilla, uva ursi
- Dandelion, gentian root (all herbs 1-2 weeks)
- + M.D.

Perspiration

Perspiration cools the body, eliminates poisons and excess heat via sweat. Too much or too little ⇨ disease.

A. Excessive, regular, profuse perspiration

General causes:

1. Summer heat, humidity, chi deficiency (CH. 4)
2. Heart disease, bacterial, viral infections, etc.

3. Diet

a) Deficient vegetables, fruit (cooling, moistening)
b) Excess protein, fat ⇨ excess weight, insulation, sweating (CH. 25, Sweaty Hands, Feet)
c) Excess coffee, alcohol, hot spices overheat

Treatment: CMD #1
• Sage tea

B. Intermittent sweating (day, night) via
• Deficient protein, fat, lack of sleep ⇨
• Weakens the lungs, skin ⇨ open pores ⇨ leak

Treatment: HMD
• Sage tea: night sweats
• +/- M.D.

C. Too little perspiration (many causes): M.D.

Pharmaceutical Drugs

Pharmaceutical drugs are an emergency medicine, both lifesaving and disease causing (side-effects), especially when multiple or long-term. Most doctors know little about these drugs aside from information (literature, sales reps) and rarely confer with one another. My father (90): **kidney doctor** recommended *calcium supplements*, **heart** doctor: *calcium blockers*. He questioned both, who said no problem. Make sense?

Case history #45. Man (65- 74), obese (20+ lbs.), clogged arteries, high blood pressure, insomnia, incontinence, difficulty walking, loss of balance. I told him it was his diet: too much animal, protein, fat, fried foods, bread, cookies, etc. He would not change. He believed, trusted his doctors (4+), multiple visits, blood work, x-rays, MRI, spinal taps, drugs, surgery, etc. that promised cures, better health. They found multiple growths, tumors (brain, spine) ⇨ surgery.

He almost died, had to be revived several times, spent two months in rehabilitation, bedridden, could not walk, had to use a wheel chair. Three months later, he could walk with a cane and walker, but still lose his balance, fall. During this time (years), he had been taking **10+ drugs** to improve cholesterol, blood pressure, urination, insomnia, walking, balance, pain (diagnosed as pre-M.S.), prostate operation (did not work). His condition progressively worsened including mood changes, anger, depression and mania.

Many of the symptoms he was experiencing were also listed **side-effects** of the prescribed drugs:

1. **Gabapentin**: anti-seizure medicine, epilepsy, pain reliever ⇨ side-effects ⇨
- Dizziness, drowsiness, tiredness, insomnia
- Clumsiness, unsteadiness, loss of balance
- Difficulty speaking, loss of strength
- Lower back pain, suicidal thoughts

2. **Prednisone**: steroid, anti-inflammatory ⇨
- Dizziness, weak muscles, moodiness, edema

3. **Amlodipine**: calcium channel blocker dilates blood vessels, improves blood flow for angina, heart disease, high blood pressure ⇨
- Low blood pressure, angina, heart attack
- Severe dizziness, light headedness, feinting

4. **Metoprolol succinate**: beta blocker for angina, hypertension ⇨
- Lightheaded feeling, feinting
- Shortness of breath

5. **Analeptic**: high BP, congestive heart failure ⇨
- Dizziness, weakness

6. **Hydrochlorothiazide**: high blood pressure or edema caused by steroids ⇨
  - Muscle weakness, dizziness

7. **Prodigal**: anticoagulant, blood thinner, prevents blood clots ⇨
   • Stomach pain, dizziness

8. **Temirtau**: high blood pressure ⇨
   • Headache, dizziness, extreme fatigue
   • Fainting, lightheadedness, chest pain

Drugs #3- 8: heart disease, blood clots, high blood pressure, arthritis: caused by poor diet. His doctors (different hospitals, locations) never questioned his diet and rarely conferred with one another, yet were always willing to treat, medicate, operate, no matter the risk, cost. He ended up in constant pain, barely able to walk (walker, wheelchair), miserable, no will to live. His last four months were spent in a hospital. He was once a vibrant, happy, outgoing, funny person. He believed in doctors, and he got worse. This was my brother. His story, unfortunately is most people's story, present and future, that can be changed. The body will heal itself when given the chance (diet, exercise, etc.). More info: CH. 9 (Circulation), 50+ case histories.

Plantar Fasciitis

Looseness, inflammation of plantar fascia (ligaments, tendons, muscles: holds, moves the bones in the feet) ⇨
   • Excruciating pain (feet, heels), especially in A.M., upon rising or after sitting, lying down long-time.

General causes:
1. Obesity, gout/ purine/ uric acid), injury
2. Excessive exercise, bad shoes

3. Diet

a) Deficient protein, fat (animal, plant) ⇨
   • Thin, deficient blood (low protein, fat) ⇨
   • Thins, dries, inflames, weakens, loosens, shakes, pains the bones, ligaments, muscles, nerves, etc.

Treatment: HMD
- Turmeric, guggul
- Avoid high purine foods, drinks (CH. 22, Gout), coffee/ caffeine

b) Excess protein sat. fat, cholesterol (animal) ⇨
- Clots, plaque ⇨ narrow, clogged arteries ⇨
- Reduced circulation, blood ⇨ legs, feet, ligaments, muscles, etc. ⇨ weak, loose, PF

Treatment: CMD #1, 2
- Vegetables (raw > cooked)
- Mild spices, bitter herbs

Case history #3. I (53) excruciating heel pain, especially upon wakening, standing, which did seem to get better with walking (increased circulation), but not cure. I thought I was doomed, and resigned to suffering what came with old age. After 7- 8 months of continual pain, limping, dragging my feet, I consulted an M.D., podiatrist: diagnosed **Plantar Fasciitis**: loose ligaments ⇨ heal pain. He recommended:
1. Surgery: cut open heels, sew, tighten ligaments
2. Orthotics
3. Hot, cold compresses

His treatment, cure seemed more like pain management than a permanent cure. I declined. His diagnosis, Plantar Fasciitis, loose ligaments, however helped me greatly, figure out the cause: narrow arteries (past high animal, fat) ⇨ reduced blood flow ⇨ feet, ligaments ⇨ loose. I switched to CMD #1, grains, vegetables, fruit, spices, horsetail, bitter herbs (golden seal, turmeric, etc.). It took **3 months** to cure: no pain whatsoever.

Plantar Fasciitis is sometimes misdiagnosed as **heel spurs** (pointed growth on heels) via heal strain, stress.

Treatment:
- Distilled water, bromelain +/- M.D.

Pneumonia

Lung infection (bacteria, viruses, fungi, inhaled food, drink or saliva) ⇨ inflame alveoli ⇨ fills: mucus, pus ⇨
- Painful breathing, coughing, chest pain
- Expectoration, hacking: mucus, phlegm
- High fever, headaches, nausea, diarrhea

General causes:

1. Weak immunity via drugs, sex, smoking, etc.

2. Obesity: excess mucus (CH. 6, Lungs)
- Mucus fosters the growth of bacteria, viruses, etc.

Treatment: CMD #2: excess mucus, obesity
- Spices, flax seeds, elecampane, marshmallow
- Golden seal, echinacea, bayberry + M.D.

Postnasal drip

Case history #46 Woman (20's): postnasal drip via cold, damp diet (soft dairy, salads, juices, cold drinks, sodas) ⇨ excess water ⇨ nose ⇨ leaks, drips. I advised cooked vegetables, spices, etc. It took two days to cure.

Premenstrual Syndrome (PMS)

Series of physical, mental symptoms associated with abnormal menstruation: early, absent or delayed, varies according to **constitution** and **diet** (CH. 16, Ayurveda).

1. Vata (air, thin, dry) or low protein, fat, high fruit, vegetables, raw, juices ⇨
- Anemia, amenorrhea (little or no period)
- Irregular, short, 3- 5 days, scanty menses
- Severe cramping, lower back pain, bloating
- Dry skin, thirst, constipation, headache
- Dizziness, feinting, mood swings, anxiety
- Worse at sunrise, sunset (vata times)

Treatment: HMD (anti-vata)
- No red meat
- Bitters: aloe vera gel, valerian, dang gui
- Turmeric, nutmeg in warm milk before bed
- +/- M.D.

2. Kapha (water) or high dairy, fat, sugar, salads, fruit, juice, cold drinks ⇨
- Menstrual flow, moderate, 7+ days
- Pale, light red blood, mucus discharge
- Swollen breasts, edema (lower legs, painful)
- Nausea, lethargy, crying, loss of appetite
- Worse early morning, evening

Treatment: CMD #2 (anti-kapha)
- Chilies, spices: black pepper, cayenne, ginger
- Bitters: turmeric, aloe vera gel
- +/- M.D.

3. Pitta (fire) or high animal, protein, fat, oil, spices, fermented foods, drinks (alcohol) ⇨
- Excessive menstrual flow (5- 7 days +/-)
- Warm, dark, red, purple blood, clots
- Diarrhea (yellow), fever, sweating, thirst
- Flushed face, red eyes, rashes, insomnia
- Joint pain, anger, irritability, short temper
- Worse at noon, midnight

Treatment: CMD #1 (anti-pitta)
- Turmeric, saffron, aloe vera, gotu kola
- +/- M.D.

Menstrual cramps:
- 1 TB aloe vera gel + ¼ tsp. black pepper 3x/ day and or valerian until cramps disappear

Prostate disease

Prostate: doughnut shaped, chestnut size male sex gland, encircles neck of urethra ⇨ stores, releases semen, prostatic fluids ⇨ penis.

PATHOLOGIES:

1. Benign prostatic hypertrophy: non-cancerous enlargement of prostate
2. Prostatitis: inflammation of prostate
3. Tumor, cancer: prostate, testicles

General symptoms:
- Frequent, urgent, interrupted, or painful urination
- Pain (perineal, lower back), fatigue
- Impotence, premature ejaculation

General causes:

1. Old age

2. Excess sex, suppression of ejaculation (CH. 16)

3. Diet: excess protein, saturated fat, cholesterol

Treatment: CMD #1, 2
- Organic beets (raw or juice), onions, garlic
- Pumpkin seeds: organic, raw, ground; parsley
- Lemon grass, uva ursi, echinacea, ashwagandha
- Saw palmetto normalizes prostate, relieves perineal pain, increases testosterone
- Echinacea (tumors), uva ursi
- Irish moss, kelp, seaweed reduces swelling
- Less or sex relaxes, strengthens prostate
- +/- M.D.

Prostate cancer (CH. 20): virtually unknown in China (low animal, high plant diet), certain areas where men eat one handful of pumpkin seeds (zinc, EFA) daily

Beets (organic, raw): oxygen, anti-cancer/ tumor
- More info: CH. 20 (Cancer). Alexander Ferenczi M.D., Department of Internal Diseases, district hospital at Csoma, late 1950's successfully treated lung and prostate cancer with beetroot.

Psoriasis

Painful skin disorder: face, scalp, ears, back, shoulders, genitalia ⇨
- Dry, red, itchy, scaly +/- flakes, dandruff
- Alternates: exacerbation, remission

General causes:
1. Toxins, chemical poisons, pollution
2. Poor diet: high protein, fat, sugar

Treatment: CMD #1
- Mild spices: cumin, coriander, fennel
- Bitters: gotu kola, dandelion, burdock, turmeric
- +/- M.D.

Case history #1. 2008 Man (38), **obese**, chronic **psoriasis** since childhood (M.D., drugs): dry, red, scaly. itchy skin, scalp, dandruff, as well as medications. Long-term diet: red meat, pork, fried foods, chips, sugar, alcohol, smoker. I advised less animal, red meat, fried foods, more fruit, vegetables, organic raw carrots (snack). He worked where I lived (retirement village). I often shopped with him, gave him advice, warnings. **Seven** months later, complete cure: 60 lb. weight loss, brand new, healthy, glowing skin, looked 15 years younger, started cooking for his family.

25. "R- S" DISEASES

Rash

Skin eruption (arms, armpits, groin, etc.): red, flat, raised, dry, oily.

General causes:

1. Alcohol, hit, damp climate, diapers, cosmetics

2. Clogged intestines, obesity, skin allergies

3. Measles, chicken pox, rubella, herpes, genetics

4. Diet: excess fat, nut butters, chips, cookies, chocolate, sugar, alcohol thickens, clogs, heats liver, gall bladder (energetic pathway, meridian passes through groin), lymph glands (groin, armpit) ⇨ hot, red, oily rashes (damp heat)

Treatment: CMD #2
- Smaller meals, cooked, raw vegetables
- Bitters: turmeric, gentian, dandelion root
- Topical:
- Turmeric cream, aloe vera gel
- Coriander: boil 1 tsp. seeds: 1 C water, 10 min.

Dietary rashes take months to develop and weeks, months to cure. Left untreated ⇨ psoriasis.

Case history #28. I (60's): red, oily, stinky rash (both armpits) via overeating, fat, sugar. I switched to the CMD #1. Right rash, armpit (liver) took two months to cure. Left armpit (spleen) more difficult, required greater discipline, time, one year to cure, in addition to my sour body odor.

Restless Leg Syndrome

Irresistible urge to move the legs +/- tingling, throbbing, numbness, shaking, twitching of ligaments tendons, muscles, especially when seated or legs raised ⇨ decreased circulation, blood (nutrients) ⇨ dries, weakens, shakes (air, wind). Water, protein, fat, minerals, etc. via blood, arteries, veins, etc. build, fuel, moisten, hold, move nerves, ligaments, bones, etc.

General causes:

1. Diet

a) Low protein, fat ⇨ extreme
•   Treatment: HMD

b) Obesity, atherosclerosis, high fat, animal, sugar
•   Treatment: CMD #1, exercise, walking

Case history #47. I (50's, clogged arteries via high protein, fat diet): numbness, pain, shaking, etc. It took one month to cure via CMD #1.

2. Injury, drugs, etc.

Shaking

Trembling (lack of holding) of limbs. Jing/ ojas (sexual essence, CH. 16) and blood (nutrients) build, fuel, moisten, hold the nerves, bones, muscles, etc.

General causes:

1. Nervous system disorder: Parkinson's, epilepsy
2. Smoking, sex, caffeine: drying

3. Diet

a) Long-term low protein, fat ⇨ thins, dries, weakens (chi deficiency: lack of holding), airs, shakes the nerves, bones, muscles, etc.

b) Excess protein, fat ⇨ narrow, clogged arteries ⇨ reduce blood ⇨ extremities, head, arms, legs

4. Winter cold ⇨ moves blood away from the head, shoulders, arms (⇨ dry, shake) to chest, abdomen: vital organs.

Treatment: HMD (2a), CMD #1 (2b) +/- M.D.

Shingles (herpes zoster)

Herpes virus, infection ⇨
- Red skin, blisters, lesions, inflamed nerves
- Chronic or intermittent pain: severe, mild
- 1 million cases/year: age 50+ (110 million, U.S.A.)

General causes:

1. Childhood measles, chicken pox

2. Diet: Excess protein, fat, caffeine, alcohol heat, dry, inflame, pain the nerves, redden the skin

Treatment: CMD #2
- Bitter herbs: chamomile, red clover
- Topical: raw honey or licorice extract: pain, sores
- +/- M.D.

Case history. Two friends. Man, woman (age 60+), overweight, high protein, fat diet: vaccinated (shingles). Two weeks later developed shingles.

Sinusitis

Inflammation of paranasal sinuses: 4 air-filled, moist (sinus secretions, mucus cleanses debris) pockets in bones around nose ⇨ connect ⇨ throat ⇨ lungs
1. **Frontal** above eyes
2. **Ethmoid** either side and above nose
3. **Sphenoid** behind bridge of nose
4. **Maxillary** inside cheekbones

General causes:

1. Smoking, pollution dries, inflames, infects
2. Diet, excess dairy, sugar, fruit, juices, sodas, cold drinks ⇨ excess water, mucus in sinuses ⇨
- Obstruction, inflammation, sinusitis

Treatment: CMD #2
- Hot spices (cayenne, black pepper, cinnamon, basil): antiviral, dry, decongest the sinuses
- Mullein, licorice: bitter, sweet, cooling, anti-inflammatory, expectorant

Case history #48. Woman (30's): sinusitis via dairy, salads, juices, cold drinks. I recommended the CMD #2, cooked vegetables, spices. It took one week to cure.

Sore Lower Back

Lower back pain can indicate:
- Kidney weakness via excess sex, cold drinks
- Injury, chronic disease, bad mattress
- Poor posture, sitting too long

Case history #49. I, sore lower back via excess ice cream, cold drinks, was cured easily: spicy soup, tea.

Sore Throat

Sore, dry, red, irritated throat, hoarse voice

General causes:
1. Smoking, hot dry climate
2. Excessive talking, yelling

Treatment:
- Gargle: coconut oil (antibacterial, anti-inflammatory) 20 minutes, ghee, sesame oil: do not swallow
- 1 TB honey in hot water
- Smokers: peppermint tea (2x/ day)

3. Congestion: mucus, phlegm

Treatment:
- Spicy vegetable soup
- Gargle 1 tsp. each: sage, bayberry (tea)

4. Flu ⇨
- Severe, swollen, infected throat: streptococcus

Treatment:
- Antibiotic: golden seal, yellow dock, echinacea
- Gargle: grape seed extract, turmeric or bayberry
- M.D., antibiotics (penicillin)

Streptococcus is extremely difficult to cure naturally. It should not be taken lightly, can result in death. More info: About the Author: case history #55.

5. Laryngitis (loss of voice): CH. 23

Sweaty Hands, Feet

Woman (40's): long-term, profuse sweating via feet, hands. Her diet: coffee, grilled cheese sandwich for breakfast; meat, rice for lunch (no fruit, vegetables) overheated her body ⇨ profuse perspiration (worse in summer). Her son (18) also had the same condition, underwent surgery (removed sweat glands in hands, feet) ⇨ cured sweating (hands, feet), but increased sweating everywhere else. I recommended more fruit, vegetables, but never saw her again.

26. "T- Z" DISEASES

Teeth

The teeth, bones, nerves and gums are built, dried, moistened, purified or rotted by food, drugs, smoking, etc. **Natural foods**: fruit, vegetables, grains, beans, nuts, seeds, juices (unsweetened) provide easily digested, assimilated **nutrients**, protein fat, minerals, etc. that build the teeth, bones, have very little residue, poisons, are easy to clean, do little damage unlike animal, processed, oily, sweet, salty foods, candies, cookies, crackers, chips, etc. ⇨ greater residue, poisons, plaque, bacteria, decay, periodontal disease.

Carbohydrate sugar (fruit, vegetables, grains, far less than cane sugar, honey, maple syrup, natural, synthetic, highly processed, etc.) feeds bacteria (plaque) ⇨ above and below gum line ⇨ acids ⇨

a) Leach, demineralize, decay teeth ⇨ cavities

b) Gums ⇨ infection, periodontal disease
- Sensitivity: hot, cold foods, drinks; dry mouth
- Gingivitis: red, swollen, bleeding gums
- Pyorrhea: inflammation of gums ⇨ pockets, abscesses, bleeding, pus, halitosis
- Loose, distended teeth

Vitamin C deficiency ⇨ bleeding gums. Smoking depletes Vitamin C, heats, dries, poisons, recedes the gums. Gargle water after smoking to moisten, cleanse. Occasional: coconut or sesame oil gargle (#5) to cleanse harmful chemicals, moisten mouth, throat.

BEST prevention, care:
1. Good diet, regular flossing, brushing: soft bristle
2. Biannual dental visits, cleanings
3. Toothpaste, mouthwash: Ayurvedic, Naturopathic
4. Water, jet cannon after meals +/-

5. Gargling:

a) Oil pulling: 1 TB coconut (antibacterial, anti-inflammatory): 15- 20 min., 3x/ week ⇨ reduces bacteria, plaque, pain, helps prevent bleeding gums, decay, infections, pyorrhea, gingivitis. Do not swallow.

b) Salt water (antiseptic): cuts (tongue, mouth)

6. Sesame seeds (organic, ground, black > brown): rejuvenative (teeth, bones), receding gums

7. Amla: cleanses mouth, strengthens teeth, helps grow gums, stops bleeding

8. Myrrh (antibiotic, antiseptic, antibacterial): loose teeth (Bhringraj), gingivitis, pyorrhea, decay

9. Peppermint oil: toothache (numbs the nerves)

10. Licorice: anti-cavity, antibacterial, reduces plaque

11. Hydrogen peroxide/ warm water (1:1+) draws infection out of tooth, pops an abscess +/-

Dental treatment:

a) Filling cavities is a band-aid approach, history repeats itself without dietary changes, as every filling ⇨ crown, root canal, extraction, implant.

b) Ticking time bombs +/-
•   Root canals ⇨ 5- 20 years ⇨ fail ⇨ bone loss, infection
•   Posts in cracked or old teeth: temporary fix

c) Implants: so far, best, most practical choice, require the most care, as there is no longer a root, nerve to absorb shock, prevent damage from downward movement: tooth ⇨ root ⇨ bone.

Raw, hard vegetables, nuts, candies, flour (cookies, pretzels, chips, etc.), etc. require harder chewing, grinding, pushing down ⇨ implant ⇨ bone ⇨ decay, pain, infection; faster, worse when low bone density (cavities, old age) or old tooth, root canal, etc.

Case History #50. 2014 after 5 years absence (fear) ⇨ dentist. I: profuse bleeding, seriously bad breath, two old crowns (root canals) broken off and what looked like severe decay in front teeth. He extracted 5 teeth; told me I had severe periodontal disease, needed gum surgery ($1600) before he could treat the decay because of the bleeding. He also said my front teeth were loose that I would probably lose all my upper teeth (he was right), which freaked me out. I did not trust him, decided against surgery. Implants were a possibility but highly expensive ($3- $6,000/ tooth). I did nothing, became seriously depressed, withdrawn, did not smile for a year. I then researched dentists, implants (internet), etc.

I went to Dr. Marco Munoz Cavallini International Dental Clinic, Costa Rica: excellent quality treatment, care, state of the art equipment, substantially lower prices, free pickup at the airport to their hotel, where clinic is located, and breakfast at their restaurant.
- 2 teeth extracted (no charge with implant)
- 3 bone grafts ($900), 1 root canal ($450)
- 5 implants ($600/ implant screw)
- 6 zirconium crowns @ $450
- Super cleaning ($50): revealed no decay on front teeth. I did not need gum surgery.
- Return trip (5 months later) for crowns

2019, **2021** ⇨ Costa Rica, same prices dentistry, hotel, etc. Five teeth (root canals): bad ⇨ extracted ⇨ implants. **2023** ⇨ Costa Rice, loose front teeth, bad, old root canals. Six teeth were extracted. I got five more implants. I was in a lot of pain, took Ibuprofen, 800 mg. every four hours for two weeks until I (vegan) changed my diet, ate Swiss cheese and the pain lessened. The next day I did not eat Swiss cheese. The pain worsened.

So, I started eating Swiss cheese every day, which eliminated the pain and need for Ibuprofen.

2024. One old tooth (root canal, posts) cracked ⇨ loose, painful with hard swelling, protrusion in gum that was not an infection (abscess) because it would not pop. I took Ibuprofen for a week. **Case history #51**: I started doing oil pulling, 20 min., 1- 2x per day. Two weeks later, all pain, swelling disappeared. The tooth eventually broke off. All three teeth (root canals, posts) failed within a year, which is why, in my opinion, posts, roots canals for old teeth are in general a bad idea. Implants: so far: no problems, except occasional gum irritation.

Thyroid disease

Thyroid gland produces thyroxin ⇨ regulates body temperature, metabolism, energy.

Deficient thyroxin ⇨ hypothyroidism ⇨
- Fatigue, cold intolerance, weight gain
- Muscle weakness, cramps, migraines
- Milky discharge (breast), painful menstruation
- Yellow orange discoloration: skin (palms, hands)
- Droopy, swollen eyes, yellow bumps (eyelid)
- Constipation, hair loss, scaly skin, insomnia
- Weak immunity, respiratory infection, depression
- Mostly women, 30- 50: menstruation, diet

The following weaken the thyroid, decrease thyroxin:

1. Drugs, fluoride, pesticides, poisons
2. Long-term low fat, high sugar, caffeine, alcohol
3. Excess dairy, juices, cold drinks ⇨ phlegm ⇨ swells thyroid, lymph nodes

Treatment: correct diet
- Kelp, Irish moss (iodine), saw palmetto
- + M.D.

4. Too little iodine, thyroid tumor, disease ⇨ goiter (swelling, front of neck). Treatment: M.D.

Tinnitus

Tinnitus: ringing in ears. TCM:

1. Loud ringing: liver disease (CH. 8), alcohol
- Treatment: CMD #1, 2 ginkgo biloba, chamomile
- +/- M.D

2. Low ringing
- Kidney yin deficiency (CH. 16)
- Anemia, wax buildup (CH. 22, Hearing)

Tumors

Neoplasm: abnormal mass, growth of cells, tissues:
- Fatty, protein: benign, malignant (cancer)
- Fibrous/ fibroid tumor (CH. 21): benign

General causes:

1. Smoking, radiation

2. Diet: excess protein, saturated fat, cholesterol

Treatment CMD #1, 2
- Raw or juice: beets, leafy greens, lettuce: high nitrates, increase blood, oxygen flow
- Sunflower, alfalfa sprouts, wheat grass, nettles
- Aloe gel, turmeric, gentian, barberry, dandelion
- Burdock root; hawthorn (abdominal tumors)
- More info: CH. 20 (Cancer)

Ulcers (gastro-intestinal)

Circumscribed lesions of mucus membrane (stomach, small intestine) formed by necrotic tissue via excess acid, enzymes, fermentation ⇨ dries, burns, bleeds, pains ⇨ red stools, vomiting blood. General causes:

1. Diet: overeating fatty, spicy, fermented foods, drinks, alcohol ⇨ excess acidity (SI, LI)

Treatment: CMD #1
- Bland diet, whole grains, milk fast
- Alfalfa, mung bean sprouts, cooked vegetables
- Herbs: licorice, marshmallow, slippery elm
- Stomach ulcers: fresh cabbage juice
- Bitters: dandelion, golden seal, licorice
- +/- M.D.

2. Diet: too little protein, fat ⇨ weak digestion ⇨ increases poisons ⇨ increases acidity

3. Deficient mucus, HCl acid, enzymes (pepsin)
- Treatment: supplement (HCl, pepsin) + M.D.

Urinary Tract Infection (UTI)

Inflammation: urinary bladder, urethra ⇨
- Difficult painful, burning urination

General causes:

1. Bacterial contamination via sex or fecal matter: women (proximity of urethra, anus)

2. Diet:

a) Excess fat, protein, spices, sour foods, wine, nightshades (tomatoes, potatoes, eggplant, etc.) ⇨ acute infections: most common

Treatment: CMD #1
- Sandalwood (anti-septic), coriander, fennel
- Cranberry, coconut, pomegranate juice+/- M.D.

b) Excess dairy, sugar (any) ⇨ excess blood sugar ⇨ feeds bacteria (UTI), yeast (genital, oral areas)

Treatment: CMD #2
- Spices: cinnamon, parsley, coriander, fennel
- Diuretics: juniper berry, gotu kola (pain) +/- M.D.

3. Vata, dryness (CH. 5): chronic, mild, irregular

Treatment: protein, fat (animal, plant)
*   Raw beets, cooked sweet round root vegetables
*   Ashwagandha, sarsaparilla, corn silk
*   +/- M.D.

Vaginitis

Inflammation of vagina ⇨ pain, itching, burning urination, yellow, foul-smelling discharge

General causes:

1. Candidiasis, UTI, sexually transmitted disease

2. Diet: excess meat, fish, eggs, cheese, fried foods, oil, sugar, alcohol

Treatment: CMD #2, aloe, horsetail +/- M.D.

Varicose Veins

Pooling of blood: veins (legs, feet) via malfunctioning valves ⇨ swollen, bulging, bluish, lumpy-looking veins, affects women > men.

General causes:
1. Sitting or standing too long, heavy lifting
2. Obesity, liver, heart disease, tumors
3. Pregnancy

Treatment: CMD #1, 2
*   Nuts, seeds (EFA), milk thistle
*   Bitters (barberry, golden seal, Butcher's broom)
*   Spices (garlic), Witch hazel (topical)
*   Wash, soak veins with apple cider vinegar
*   +/- M.D.

*   Acupuncture lances, bleeds varicose veins

Venereal disease

Treatment: vegetarian diet
- Herpes (CH. 22): aloe vera, sarsaparilla, gotu kola
- Syphilis: golden seal, gonorrhea: myrrh
- + M. D.

Vision

Poor vision, seeing floaters, constant blinking. Nutrients via diet via blood, circulation, capillaries, arteries, veins, heart ⇨ build, fuel, moisten the eyes.

General causes:

1. Diet

a) Deficient protein, fat weakens, twitches eyelids

Treatment: HMD (no red meat)
- Carrot tops/ greens (raw, organic): high Vitamin A (CH. 2): see following case history
- Raw or juices: beets, leafy greens, lettuce
- Valerian, amla, licorice

b) Excess protein, saturated fat, cholesterol ⇨
- Narrow, clogged coronary arteries ⇨ reduces blood, nutrients, protein, EFA, oxygen, etc. ⇨ head ⇨ eyes ⇨ weaken, dry
- Bumps, growths (protein) on eyelids

Treatment: CMD #1, 2
- Raw vegetables, organic carrot tops
- Ashwagandha, valerian
- Chrysanthemum, eye-bright, bilberry: improves vision, brightens eye
- Nettles (puffy eyes)

Case history #51. My vision (54) started going bad, which forced me to buy reading, magnifying glasses.

Despite eating organics carrots (high Vitamin A) without tops, said to improve vision) for the last 30 years, my vision was still going bad. One day, while shopping I (lacto-vegetarian, spices, etc.). decide to buy raw, organic **carrots with tops**. A few months later, my vision improved. I could now read most of the time without glasses. Age 73, driver's license vision test: 20:20. I healed quickly because for many years I had been eating a vegetarian diet, organic and exercising regularly (improves arteries, circulation, blood to eyes).

2. Excess radiation: TV, computer (modified screens reduce glare), etc. especially at night weakens

3. Sex, old age, smoking dries, weakens

4. Sitting on lower legs, bent underneath the buttocks: common in Japan, China, etc., weakens the eyes. Many Asians wear glasses.

5. Night blindness via Vitamin A deficiency
   • Treatment: organic carrots + tops (raw), Vit. A supplement: food based

6. Macular degeneration: spinach

7. Conjunctivitis: chamomile (decoction/ tea, wash), aloe, barberry

Crying moistens the eyes.

Bates Method exercise: looking up, down, left, right, circling in both directions 6- 12x each strengthens.

Worms

Infestation of worms in small intestine via raw foods (plant, animal +/- quality, etc.) ⇨
1. Hookworms: desire to eat strange objects (wax, soil, uncooked rice, tea leaves)
2. Round worms: vomited

3. Pinworms: itchy anus, worse in evening
4. Tapeworms: constant hunger
- All: abdominal pain, distention, cold limbs

Treatment: CMD #2
- Cayenne, aloe vera gel
- Round, pinworms: chamomile
- Round, pin, tapeworms: pomegranate, garlic
- +/- M.D.

Yeast infection

Excess yeast (fungi), Candida ⇨ vagina

General dietary causes:

a) Excess water, sugar, yeast via dairy, bread, juice, sodas ⇨ blood ⇨ uterus, vagina ⇨
- Thick, white, watery, milky, clumpy discharge
- White flakes, infection (UTI), itching, burning

Treatment: CMD #2
- Cabbage juice, sage tea, caprylic acid
- Hot spices, prickly ash; mugwort (douche)
- Astringent: raspberry leaf, mullein
- Vinegar douche, inserting garlic clove in vagina
- +/- M.D.

b) Excess fat, meat, fish, eggs, whole dairy, sugar, alcohol ⇨ blood ⇨ uterus, vagina, kidneys ⇨
- Infection, yellow discharge, burning urination

Treatment: CMD #2
- Cabbage juice, sage tea, caprylic acid
- Mild spices: fennel, coriander, turmeric
- Raspberry leaf, damiana
- Bitters: myrrh, golden seal, mullein
- +/- M.D.

Case history #52. I (health food store) met many women: cured yeast infections via diet, herbs.

Section III. Daily Practices

27. WAY OF BREATHING

The body (30 trillion cells) is 70% water (like earth), 65% oxygen (O_2). Oxygen is a vital nutrient, water-soluble gas that enlivens, electrifies, protects, purifies, kills viruses, cancer, etc. A few minutes without ⇨ cellular death, especially brain, heart. The brain uses 30%. The lungs control the breath, air, respiration:
1. Inhale, take in oxygen via green plants, trees
2. Eliminate carbon dioxide (CO_2): cellular waste product: protein, starch, sugar

Breathing exercises, fresh air, oxygen improve the blood, lungs, heart, circulation, elimination, immunity, relax the mind and are commonly used in meditation (CH. 30), chi gung (CH. 28), yoga and martial arts.

Poor diet, posture, inactivity, smoking, vaping, sadness weakens the lungs, decreases energy, vitality.

Five ways to breathe:

1. **Chest**
- Rib cage expands, draws in, fills, and contracts, empties only the top third of lungs ⇨
- Less O_2 absorbed, more CO_2 retained ⇨
- Rapid breathing to increase O_2, eliminate CO_2
- Shallow, inefficient

2. **Abdominal**
- Practice: indoors, outdoors, standing, sitting or lying on one's back
- Efficient, uses entire capacity of lungs

a) Inhalation: nose ⇨ throat ⇨ stomach, fill, expand, push out abdomen ⇨ lower ⇨ middle ⇨ upper ⇨ draws air, O_2 deeper ⇨ lungs from bottom ⇨ top

- Hold 5- 10 seconds (do not strain) ⇨ greater absorption. Straining, holding too long can harm the lungs and induce unconsciousness.

b) Exhalation ("**ha**" sound): mouth via contraction, pushing in abdomen: bottom ⇨ middle ⇨ top ⇨ expels more CO_2. Relax 5 seconds

c) Repeat: 20 minutes +/-

3. **Embryonic**
- How the fetus breathes inside the womb, via the umbilicus

a) Inhalation: nose via contraction of the abdomen (pushes in) with inhalation ⇨ front ⇨ side ⇨ rear

b) Exhalation: mouth, nose via expansion of the abdomen (pushes out) in the same order

c) Repeat #a, b: 20 minutes +/-

4. **Pranayama breathing**
- Deep abdominal (#2): inhalation held (5- 10 seconds +) then exhalation 2x (20 seconds +/-).
- Best done: outdoors (fresh air), early, late morning or evening (stars)
- Practice: 20 min. +/-
- Caution: too much prana, without the proper amount of ojas (CH. 5) overexcites, heats, weakens ⇨ insomnia.

Abdominal breathing #2- 4 increases:
- Energy, quiets, relaxes the mind
- Longevity via lesser breaths. Taoism: everyone is given a certain number of breaths. When those breaths expire, death ensues. Most people breathe 10x per minute. Slowing: 5- 7x/ minutes uses less energy, extends life.

Do not practice abdominal breathing if:
a) Smoker (includes vaping): poisonous chemicals (tobacco: 100+, marijuana): kill lung cells, contract, dry tissues, blood ⇨ tumors, cancer
- Abdominal breathing draws toxins deeper into LG

b) Lung damage can be reversed, cleansed (months – 30+ years, depending on severity) via diet, circulation of blood and cessation of smoking. More info: **Case history #19** (CH. 6): 80-year-old man, smoked for 40+ years, stopped at age 60, now has healthy lungs: no traces of smoke or damage, verified by his pulmonary doctor, x-rays.

c) Pregnant, menstruating: abdominal breathing creates downward pressure on uterus, sex organs

d) Live in a polluted environment, lung disease

The following breathing exercise is used in yoga and meditation.

5. **Alternate nostril**
* Balances the flow of energy, prana ⇨ brain via
* **Ida** and **pingala**: two of three energy channels (nadis) that supply prana to the body.
* Start at base of spine ⇧ alongside right, left ⇧ brain
* Body: 72,000 nadis

a) **Ida** (left)
* Connects ⇨ **left nostril** ⇨ controls **right** brain ⇨
* Moon energy, feminine, feeling, intuition
* Cools, moistens, soothes
* Promotes sleep, dreams, imagination
* Excess breathing: left nostril ⇨ depression, anxiety, excessive sleep

b) **Pingala** (right)
* Connects ⇨ **right nostril** ⇨ controls **left** brain ⇨
* Sun energy, masculine, reason, rationality
* Excess breathing: right nostril ⇨ hyperactivity, insomnia, dizziness, anger, criticism

Practice (20 min. +/-): use thumb and forefinger to alternate, open, close the nostrils, direct breath.
1. Inhale: left nostril (close right)
2. Exhale: right (close left)

3. Inhale: right (close left)
4. Exhale: left (close right)
5. Repeat #1- 4

Balanced breathing ⇨ health, calmness, greater control, lucidity. Imbalance ⇨ disease, excess, deficiency.
- To correct imbalance, breath more through opposite nostril.
- Anger, hyperactivity, hypertension: breathe through left nostril.

Additional pranic breathing exercises
- **Yoga and Ayurveda** David Frawley

Chinese medicine: heaven's (stars) and earth's force (energy) interact, create the body.
1. Heaven's force moves down ⇩ head (crown) ⇩ brain ⇩ neck ⇩ spine ⇩ legs ⇩ feet ⇩
2. Earth's force rises ⇧ feet ⇧ legs, hips, spine ⇧ head

Heaven's force ⇨ 8 extraordinary meridians (energetic pathways, reservoirs, distribute qi, blood) ⇨
a) 12 regular, organ meridians ⇨
b) 15 branches ⇨ 12 muscle, 12 skin regions
• Acupuncture: each meridian, branch specific energy points: regulate organs, muscles, etc.

Du, Ren: two major extraordinary meridians ⇨ originate: lower abdomen ⇨ exit ⇨ perineum (midway: urethral opening, scrotum and anus) ⇨

1. Du ⇧ up back, along the spine ⇧ neck ⇧ middle, top of head ⇩ down forehead ⇩ mouth (roof)
• Feeds yang organs: GB, UB, LI, SI, ST, TB

2. Ren ⇧ up front, abdomen ⇧ neck ⇧ mouth (roof)
• Feeds yin organs: LV, K, SP, HT, LG, P

Touching tongue to roof of mouth connects Du, Ren.

12 organ meridians (CH. 4) pass up, down ⇔ head, spine via abdomen, chest, arms, legs, hands, feet.

Arms, hands, fingers:
• Heart (HT), Pericardium (P): protective sac (HT)
• Small (SI), large intestine (LI), Lungs (LG)
• Triple burner (TB): chest (circulation, respiration), upper abdomen (digestion), lower abdomen (reproduction, elimination)

Legs, feet, toes:
• Spleen (SP), stomach (ST), gall bladder (GB)
• Liver (LV), kidneys (K), urinary bladder (UB)

Every time you move, twist, turn or bend the head, chest, abdomen, back, arms, legs, spine you stimulate the related meridians, organs, glands, functions, etc.

Chi, prana is super, far more powerful than muscular energy. Real life stories:

1. **East**: Bill Moyer's television special (PBS) on China, chi gung and martial arts. There was one line of 12 men standing, front ⇨ back pushing forward into one into another into the chest of a standing **80-year-old** man (chi gung master) who did not move until a few seconds later when he appeared to lower, sink, then suddenly straighten up and thrust out his abdomen, which forcibly threw the 12 men back through the air. Paramahansa Yogananda also performed the same feat.

2. **West**: scared young, thin 100-pound mother is suddenly able to lift a 2,000# car off her child.

Chi gung (energy work): series of exercises that control, direct and hold energy within the body, include many yogic and martial arts exercises. General rules:
1. Empty stomach: minimum 2 hrs. after meal
2. Outdoors or on wooden floor
3. Early morning or late evening (negative ions)
4. Total practice: 20 minutes +

Chi Gung #1 Standing Exercise (Tree)

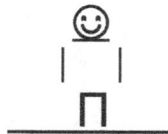

☺
| |
Π
_____

Basic chi gung exercise (**horse** stance) for channeling heavens and earth's force, like a tree.
• Body: erect, deeply rooted, strong, flexible
• Practice beginning, end, 5 minutes +/-

Posture, imagination:

1. **Head** is held, as if suspended from a string attached to the crown.

2. **Tongue** connects, touches the roof of the mouth

3. **Chin** tucked in: straightens the neck, aligns the 7 cervical vertebrae, spinal column bones: 8 cervical nerves. Relax, sink one vertebra at a time from top to bottom.

4. **Shoulders** pulled back, chest out, stomach in

5. **Spine** 12 thoracic, 5 lumbar nerves, vertebrae. Consciously relax, let body weight sink, one vertebra at a time, top to bottom.

6. **Hips** 5 sacral nerves, vertebra. The hips are tilted in to straighten the lower spine

7. **Knees** slightly bent, extend directly over, but not beyond the toes ⇨ can injure the knees.

8. **Legs** shoulder's width apart. Body weight evenly distributed left, right, front, back, heels, balls of **feet**, parallel or slightly pointed outwards.

9. **Arms, hands** hang loose, down near outside of thighs, out in front, like holding a beach ball, fingers, tips point to each other, barely touch
   - Parallel with chest: circulation, respiration
   - Below ribs: digestion
   - Below navel: reproduction, elimination

10. **Eyes** slightly opened or fully closed.

11. Imagine, feel heaven's force move down ⇨ crown, head, neck, spine, back of legs, through the feet, feeling the body sink, root into the ground.

12. Feel earth's energy rise up ⇧ feet ⇧ legs ⇧ spine ⇧ head. Relax (10 sec.). Repeat 5- 10X.

13. Breathe slowly, quietly, abdominally (CH. 27), relax 5+ minutes, empty the mind of all thoughts

Standing tree posture, rooting: one of the most powerful chi gung exercises, can be done alone (20+ minutes). It does not, however stretch, bend or twist the body, which is why additional exercises are performed.

Chi Gung #2 Look Left, Look Right

1. **Horse stance** with arms relaxed, hanging loosely at the sides. The eyes look straight ahead. Relax.

2. **Inhale** deeply, slowly into lower abdomen ⇨
3. **Exhale**, slowly turn head (chin parallel to shoulders) to the left, stare over left shoulder (few sec.) ⇨
4. **Inhale**, turn back to center or bend head forward, down (exhale), up, backwards (inhale) ⇨
5. **Exhale**, turn head slowly to right, stare over shoulder (benefits eyes, liver). Hold few seconds, inhale, return.
6. Repeat 6- 12 times

This exercise increases blood, chi ⇨ head, brain. It mimics the head movements of turtle (lives 100 yrs.+)

Chi Gung #3 Adjusting the Triple Burner

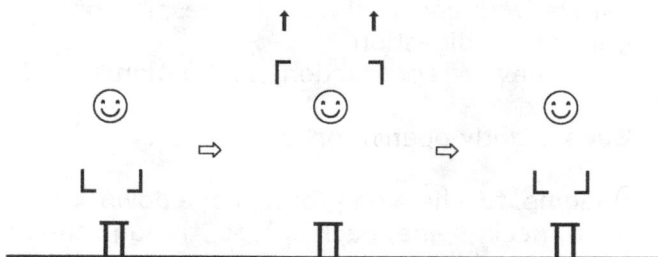

1. **Horse stance** hands, fingertips close (separate or interlaced), palms facing up 3" below navel
2. **Inhale** slowly, deeply into the abdomen. With breath, raise arms, hands, palms facing up ⇨ out, up ⇨ arc over the head ⇨ hands, palms face, push up. The head, eyes stare straight then follow the hands as they pass the eyes. Hold: few seconds.
3. **Exhale**, slowly with exhalation lower hands, arms, rotating the palms down (eyes follow until level) back to their original position.
4. Repeat 6- 12x

This exercise moves chi, stimulates triple b. (CH. 4).

Chi Gung #4 Uniting Fire and Water

1. Raise the chi   2. Lower the chi

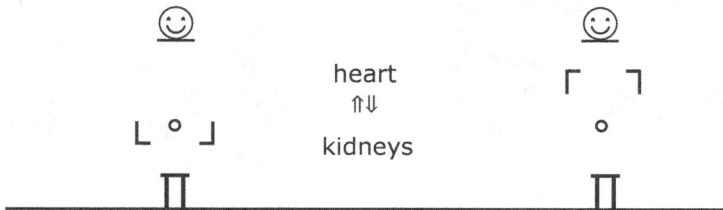

```
        ☺                                    ☺

                       heart          ┌     ┐
                        ⇑⇓
      ∟ ° ⌋                              °
                      kidneys
        ∏                               ∏
```
_____

1. **Horse stance** hands 3" below navel, palms up, fingertips pointing towards one another.
2. **Inhale** deeply, slowly into abdomen, while raising the hands, palms, directing the breath (chi) up the body (like an elevator) lower ⇨ middle ⇨ upper abdomen ⇨ chest, slightly above solar plexus (below sternum). Hold the breath.
3. Turn the palms over, **exhale** push, direct the breath, chi down ⇨ lower abdomen. Relax.
4. Repeat 6- 12x.

This exercise moves chi up, down, unites fire (heart) and water (kidneys, jing), also moves food, stools down.

Chi Gung #5 Adjust Stomach and Spleen

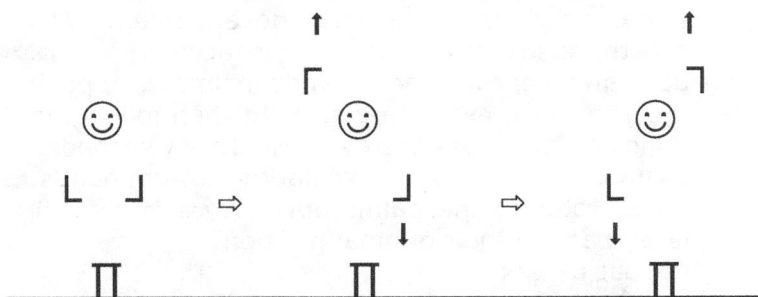

1. **Horse stance** with hands, palms up, three inches below the navel, fingertips almost touching

2. **Inhale** deeply, slowly. At the same time slowly raise the **right** arm and rotate the hand, palm in an arc up and away from the body until it passes the eyes, at which time the hand, palm rotates up over the head pushes up when fully extended. **Left** hand, palm rotates, faces, pushes down. Hold (few seconds). Exhale, reverse, lower right arm, rotate right hand down and left hand up back to their original positions.

3. Do the reverse. The **left** arm, hand, palm rises, while the **right** hand, palm pushes down. Hold. Exhale, return hands to original positions.

Repeat 6- 12x. This exercise stretches the abdomen, stimulates the spleen, stomach, moves energy, food, wastes down, helps relieve bloating, constipation.

Chi gung #6 Turning the Waist

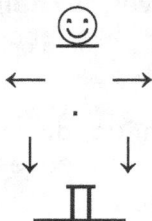

1. **Horse stance** arms at sides or hands on hips
- Hips, knees, legs face forward, do not turn, twist
- Upper body, not the hips twists, turns at the waist

2. Inhale slowly into lower abdomen
3. Exhale, turn upper body slowly with the breath to the right. The head, eyes look straight ahead. Hold for a few seconds.
4. Inhale, return to the center. Repeat to the left.
- This is one complete rotation.
5. Repeat 6- 12x.

This exercise stimulates the kidneys.

Chi Gung #7 Bend forward, Bend Backward

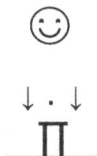

☺

↓ · ↓

Ⅱ

1. **Horse stance** arms relaxed, hang down alongside thighs, knees slightly bent. The back is help up, straight, shoulders pulled back, head slightly raised.

2. **Inhale** slowly, then **exhale**, bend over slowly with the breath from lower ⇨ middle ⇨ upper back, one vertebra at a time until fully bent over. Shoulders, neck relax as they move closer to legs.

3. **Grab** ankles, toes or balls of feet (kidney acupuncture point: bubbling wells) and pull head, body towards the knees, between the legs if flexible. Do not strain. Relax: 5- 10 seconds.

4. **Inhale**, raise the back, spine from lower ⇨ upper, vertebra by vertebra until upright. Place hands on lower back (for support), **exhale**, lean backwards. **Inhale**, return to starting position.

5. Repeat 6- 12 times.

This exercise opens the lower back, increases circulation (blood, energy), benefits the kidneys, increases flexibility.

Chi Gung #8 Lifting the Heals

1. **Horse stance**, arms hang down, relaxed

2. **Inhale** slowly raise heals (with pace of breath) off the ground. Stand on balls of feet: activates ⇨ "Bubbling wells": kidneys major acupuncture point, where earth's force enters the body (also heel, perineum). Hold a few seconds.
3. **Exhale** and slowly lower the heals (with breath) back to the ground.
4. Repeat 6- 10x.

This exercise stimulates the kidneys.

End where you began: standing, horse stance. Relax, gather chi, stand, root for 5- 10 minutes.

Chi gung can be done by young or old when healthy. **Do not practice** in the wind or rain; pregnant, physically inured, etc. Consult an M.D.

For greater instruction: teacher, classes, books or videos. Success comes with training. Practice, practice, practice. Highly recommended:
*   **Five Animal Chi Gung** by Ken Cohen (video)
*   **Taoist Eight Treasures** by Maoshing Ni (video)
*   **Eight Pieces of Brocade** by Dr. Yang Jwing Ming
*   **Beginning Chi Gung** by S. Kuei and S. Comee
*   **Opening the Energy Gates** by B. K. Frantzis: simple chi gung (kung) exercises, including standing, "tree" exercise.

"A moving gate gathers no rust." Exercise, walk daily if you want to avoid arthritis.

29. SPIRITUAL PRACTICE

Life is body, mind and spirit (Spirit). Each is a vehicle, machine, specific parts, structures, functions, physical, mental, spiritual powers, pleasures and pains via specific foods, herbs, poisons, exercises, thoughts, etc.

The purpose of this chapter and next is not spiritual indoctrination, just additional information via Ayurveda (Hinduism) about the body's spiritual structures, functions, powers, pleasures, maintenance plan.

Spirit (God) created, became the universe, all living things. "Know ye not, that ye are the temple of God and that the Spirit of God dwelleth in you." Corinthians 3:16. "Ye are gods." Psalm 82.6, **New Testament**.

Hinduism, Christianity:

A. Spirit, Cosmic Consciousness, God (**Father**) ⇨

B. Christ Consciousness (**Son**): cosmic intelligence, love, vibration of consciousness ⇨

C. Prana (cosmic life-force) ⇨ sound and light ⇨ **word** (vibratory sound, materializing power)
- Aum, Amen, Amin, **Holy Ghost**, Comforter, Divine Mother (God as nature) ⇨ material world
- "These things saith the Amen, the faithful and true witness, the beginning of creation of God" (Rev. 3:14) ⇨

Body ⇨ **brain, spine** ⇨

1. Three main energy channels (**nadis**) ⇨
- Sushumna: center of spine ("narrow is the gate")
- Ida (along left-side of spine) ⇨ left nostril ⇨ right brain ⇨ parasympathetic nervous system
- Pingala (right) ⇨ right nostril ⇨ left brain, sympathetic nervous system

2. **Kundalini**: feminine, divine energy of spiritual development, gathers, coiled at base of spine.
- Activated by prana via breathing exercises (CH. 27), meditation ⇨ rises ⇨ Sushumna ⇨ activates, purifies chakras ⇨ profound spiritual growth

3. **Chakras**: seven spiritual energy centers

North

```
  ⊛
⊖ ⊛ ⊖
 ---
```

Right		Left
	↓ ↑	
THYROID, THROAT	⊛	THYROID, TRACHEA
LUNG, THYMUS	⊛	HEART, LUNG
LIVER, GALL BLADDER SMALL INTESTINE	⊛	STOMACH, PANCREAS SPLEEN, SM. INT.
ADRENAL, OVARIES KIDNEYS, U. BLAD, LI	⊛ ⊛	ADRENAL, TESTES KIDNEY, LARGE INT.

South

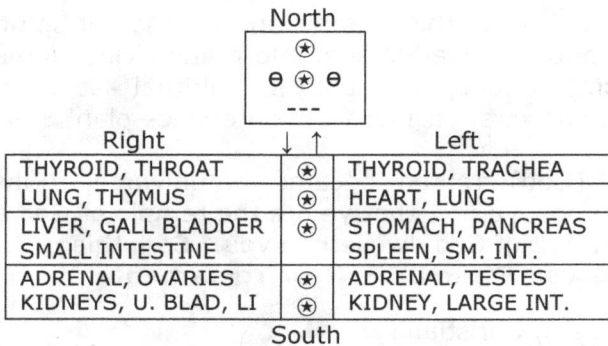

7th **Crown chakra** 1,000 pedaled lotus, throne of God, Cosmic Consciousness (kingdom of heaven, promised land, Garden of Eden), sits atop the skull
- Stores, distributes Cosmic prana to chakras
- Pineal gland (unique to humans)
- Sound: Aum, Amen: creative (A), preservative (U) and dissolutive (M) sound of all matter
- "The kingdom of God is within you." Luke17:21*

6th **Mind chakra** (3rd eye, morning star of the East): brain, frontal lobe, midway between eyebrows, connects to medulla oblongata (base of brain stem, mouth of God), where the soul enters. Three wise men of East: gold, incense, myrrh: Hinduism (wedding gifts).
- Gateway to Krishna/ Christ Consciousness ⇨ union with God, "I and my Father are one."
- Pituitary gland, nerves; sound: Aum, Amen
- Color, form: brilliant white, silvery star surrounded in circle of blue, outer yellow glow
- "Man shall not live by bread alone, but by every word (prana, sound) that proceedeth out of the mouth of God." Matt 4:4, **New Testament***

- "The light of the body is the eye, if therefore thine eye be single thy whole body shall be full of light." Matt 6:22, **New Testament**

Everyone (soul, seed of God) has Christ Consciousness ("I am the way"), divine powers and pleasures that await to be awakened via spiritual practice. "I say unto you, He that believeth on me the works that I do shall he do also, and greater works than these shall he do." John 14:12, **New Testament**.

5th **Cervical chakra**: throat (base)
- Divine calmness, intuition, expansion
- Thyroid gland, mouth, throat, respiration
- Sense: hearing, ears
- Sound: soft wind through trees, rushing water
- Color: smoky gray with little specks of light
- Ether: ability to live off cosmic energy

Therese Neumann (1898- 1962) well-documented (24-7, physicians) saint (Germany) did not eat solid food nor sleep last 40 years of her life. **Therese Neumann, Mystic and Stigmatist** by Vogl, Adalbert Albert. Also: Saint Lidwina of Schiedam, Blessed Elizabeth of Rent, Saint Nicholas of Flue, St. Catherine of Siena, etc.

4th **Dorsal chakra**: chest
- Divine love, creativity, heart
- Thymus gland, sense (touch), skin, hands
- Sound: deep gong bell
- Color: deep red or green
- Air: ability to levitate

3rd **Lumbar chakra**: umbilicus (navel)
- Determination, self-control, patience
- Pancreas gland, digestion, solar plexus, muscles
- Sense: sight, eyes; color: dark blue or yellow
- Sound: harp "I heard a voice from heaven, as the voice of many waters, and as the voice of a great thunder: and I heard the voice of harpers harping with their harps." Rev. 14:2
- Fire: walk on hot coals without burning

2nd **Sacral chakra**: 3- 4" below umbilicus
- Discipline, adherence to virtue, goodness
- Adrenal glands, reproduction, urination, bones
- Sense: taste, tongue; color: bright red/ orange
- Sound: flute, crickets; water (walk)

1st **Root chakra** (coccyx)
- Solidifies primary life-force into atoms, flesh
- Restraint, resistance to temptation, evil
- Organs of elimination: kidneys, LI, UB
- Sense: smell, nose; color: deep red
- Sound: beating drums, humming of honeybees
- Earth: become intensely heavy, immovable

Activating the chakras (stars, churches, candle sticks), kundalini, achieving Christ Consciousness, union with God: Christianity (spiritual marriage), Hinduism (Self-Realization) requires intense, long-term spiritual practice, guidance and attunement with a God-realized master, guru (Jesus, Krishna, Buddha, Moses, etc.), who are forever alive.

"The guru is the awakened God, awakening the sleeping God within the disciple." Paramahansa Yogananda (PY), **Second Coming of Christ**, page 567

"A guru's only interest is to help you progress spiritually. If the teacher wants something from the disciple, he is not a master, whose only desire is to give, not to take." PY, **Journey to Self-Realization**, p. 235

Hinduism: 4 main spiritual practices, yogas:
1. **Bhakti**: love, devotion to God, all people
2. **Karma**: action: God alone, no thought of reward
3. **Gyana**: wisdom via discrimination, study, knowledge of true Self (God)
4. **Raja** (royal): meditation, inner awareness

All include general practices: kindness, generosity, prayer (talking to God), morality, celibacy, purity, vegetarianism, etc. ⇨ help, keep, direct **energy within**, **up** the spine ⇨ brain, higher chakras ⇨ happiness, peace.

Energy down ⇨ lower three chakras, out the body ⇨ society, material world ⇨ misery, suffering.

Spiritual success, Christ Consciousness is extremely hard to do in one, much less 100 or thousand life-times, which is why God gives unlimited chances, multiple lives, incarnations and guidance (intuition, books) to get it right, overcome earthly attachment, but does not spare the rod, results, extra lives, pains of wrong thoughts, actions (karma).

Reincarnation: common belief among Christians and Jews. "Some say that thou art John the Baptist: some, Elijah; and others, Jeremiah, or one of the prophets." Matthew 16:14, New Testament.

"Him that overcometh will I make a pillar in the temple of my God, and he shall go out no more..." To him that overcometh will I grant to sit with me, in my throne, even as I also overcame, and am set down with my Father, in his throne." John, Rev. 3:12, 21, **New T.**

"Any soul who forgets its spiritual status during its earthly sojourn, forms material attachments, and thus has to reincarnate until the mundane desires are worked out and the lost divine consciousness is regained." P. Yogananda, **The Second Coming of Christ**, page 1372

"Be not deceived, God is not mocked: for whatsoever a man soweth (action), that shall he also reap (reaction). For he that soweth to the flesh shall of the flesh reap corruption; but he that soweth to the Spirit shall of the Spirit reap life everlasting." Gal. 6:7-8, New Testament

Final success is granted by the grace of God, who judges according to love. "A person who considers himself an **atheist** may sometimes, in fact, be closer to God, because of his love for other people, than many who believe in God with their minds, but whose actions towards their fellowman are uncharitable. God again watches people's deeds, not their words." Paramahansa Yogananda, **The Essence of Self-Realization**, p. 117

Reincarnation was outlawed, removed from Christian Scriptures by Emperor Justinian, Counsel of Constantinople (553 A.D.).

The following authors, books, quotes via Hinduism and Taoism help reveal the mind of God.

Paramahansa Yogananda

1. Bhagavad-Gita

"In every being there exists a masculine and feminine nature. The masculine or positive side reveals itself as the powers of discrimination, self-control, exacting-judgment-qualities that express or respond to reason. The negative or feminine nature consists of feeling-love, sympathy, kindness, mercy, joy. In the ideal being, these two aspects are perfectly balanced. But if reason lacks feeing, it becomes calculating, harsh, judgmental; if feeling lacks reason, it becomes blind emotion." p. 40

2. Revelations of Christ

"Jesus did not come on earth to show how great he was. He came to show us how great we ourselves are, in our divine potential." page 321

3. Second Coming of Jesus Christ

"Life is materialized consciousness. All consciousness comes from God." page 624

"Inner purity, not outer observances are the gauge of one's spirituality." page 856

"But by moral discipline, continuous devotional prayer, and deep meditation, God can be contacted in inner silence as Ever New Joy." page 1310

"Spirituality begins with the effort to place the well-being of someone else above one's own interests." p 1400

"To give a slap for a slap is human behavior; to give kindness for slaps is godliness." page 1451

4. **Man's Eternal Quest**

"It is when you persistently, selflessly perform every action with love-inspired thoughts of God that He will come to you. Then you will realize you are the Ocean of Life, which has become the tiny wave of each life... But greater than activity, devotion or reason is meditation. To meditate truly is to concentrate solely on the Spirit. It is the highest activity that man can perform, and it is the most balanced way to find God." page 7

5. **The Divine Romance**

"When Cosmic Consciousness comes into the realm of matter - into each of the atoms that make up the planets and island universes, and the different form of plant, animal, and human life – that Consciousness is called Christ Consciousness. When Christ Consciousness descends into the soul and pure mind of man, it is called super consciousness. Super consciousness descends into the realm of imagination; it is called subconsciousness. When subconsciousness descends into the muscular and sensory phase of human life, it is called human or waking consciousness. When waking consciousness becomes attached to the senses and material things, it is called worldly consciousness, and when it is used to harm oneself or others, it is evil consciousness. But when it is used to do good things and to produce attunement with God, then it is called spiritual consciousness." page 83

"Truths are not truths to you, unless you realize them within yourself" page 85

"Good and evil are not the creation of man, but virtue and sin are. They result from your acceptance of either good or evil." page. 92

"We should envy no one. Let others envy us. What we are, no one else is. Be proud of what you have and what you are. No one else has a personality just like yours. No one else has a face like yours. No one else has a soul like yours. You are a unique creation of God. How proud you should be!" page 390

6. Journey to Self- Realization

"Without the internal perception of God, it is very difficult to love Him. But when that Supreme Happiness permeates your thoughts and whole being, you cannot help loving Him." p. 371

"When the desire for self-interest is gone completely from the consciousness, and the only desire is to serve others and do the highest good for all, that is wisdom. It is very difficult to do; but when selfish love completely goes, then one tastes divine love." page 384

"Saints are sinners that never gave up."

Taoist Master Ni, Hua Chin

The Book of Changes and Unchanging Truth (I Ching)

"Virtuous inheritance is more important than material inheritance." page 15

"The more you eat, the less you control yourself." 360

"Flexibility, softness, calmness, and patience provide hope in a dangerous situation." page 367

"For a wise person, adversity and frustration actually become fertile soil for spiritual growth." page 495

"People who seek happiness from others, or who seek only to please others, will never discover their fountain of joy within." page 564

Learn God from the best: Jesus, Krishna, saints (men, women) of all true religions throughout the ages who have proven man's highest potential, supernatural powers, walked on water, healed the sick, raised the dead, etc., while remaining forever joyous, humble, charitable, loving to God, all despite disease, pain, hunger, homelessness, persecution, etc.

More info:
1. **Imitation of Christ** Thomas A. Kempis
2. **Mystics and Miracles** Bert Ghezzi
3. **God's Fool, The Life and Times of Francis of Assisi** Julian Green
4. **The Interior Castle** Teresa of Avilla

"By thinking of great men, women you can receive their vibrations." Paramahansa Yogananda

Author's experience: I am more confident, joyful and peaceful in their thoughts, words, than my own, which have not produced lasting happiness, just endless excuses.

You cannot change yesterday, but can change today, which changes tomorrow, for better or worse. It is not how you start, but how you finish, how much you are willing to sacrifice for God that matters.

A friend recently wished me, "Happy Birthday old man." I replied, "I am not old. It is the packaging that has gotten old."

We are not the same, but all the same.

30. MEDITATION

Meditation: deep, continual thought, focus on breath, mantras (spiritual sounds, words), brain, spine, chakras, organs, God, etc. ⇨
- Deep relaxation, inner calmness, no thought
- Supernatural powers, healing, prescience
- God-communion, never-ending joy
- Neuroplasticity: changing the brain, eliminating past imprints, brain grooves, chains of negative events, memories ⇨ replaced with new, positive thoughts, grooves ⇨ better, healthier habits.

This chapter will highlight three meditations via visualization, control, focus of energy and breath within the body, organs, meridians, brain, spine, chakras.

General requirements:

1. Healthy body, nervous system. Meditation increases energy, voltage. An unhealthy body cannot tolerate ⇨ restlessness, nerve damage.
a) Healthy diet. Vegetarian: cooling, calming
b) Meat, sugar, alcohol, drugs, overeating, sex, heat, excite, irritate, poison, tense the body, decrease will power, spiritual focus, desire.

2. Empty stomach: minimum two hours after meal

3. Physical relaxation, loose clothing, fresh air, trees

4. Silence, quietude (+/- ear plugs). Early A.M., late P.M.: best, negatively-charged times and quiet

5. Upright posture: chest out, shoulder blades pulled back, drawn slightly together, chin parallel to ground, relaxes, straightens spine ⇨ smooth energy flow ⇧⇩ brain, spine.

6. Sitting: ideal position to relax, straighten spine ⇨ improves energy flow in the spine.

a) Floor: cushion (4- 6" thick: elevates hips above knees) on woolen blanket. Legs comfortably crossed +/- full or semi lotus. No strain.

b) Chair: seat covered with woolen blanket (shields body from earth's energy pull), level with knees, feet flat on the floor, legs shoulders width apart. Back straight, do not slump forward or lean back.

7. Hands (thumb, index fingers touch), palms up or together on lap (fingers laced, thumbs touching).

Meditation: general practice time (20 minutes +/-), begin with deep abdominal breathing (3 minutes)

1. **Five clouds** (colors)

Five major organs (CH.15) control all structure function, have specific colors that nourish, cleanse.

1. Eyes closed. **Inhale**, imagine breath "bright yellow cloud" ⇨ nose ⇨ cleanses **spleen** (behind left rib cage). Hold 10 sec. +/-. **Exhale** (10 sec.) dirty yellow air. Relax. Repeat: 4 minutes ⇨

2. Lungs: bright white **in**, dirty white **out** ⇨ 4 ⇨

3. Kidneys: bright black **in**, dirty gray **out** ⇨ 4 ⇨

4. Liver: bright green **in**, dull, dark green **out** ⇨ 4 ⇨

5. Heart: bright red **in**, dull, dark red **out** ⇨ 4

II. **Du, Ren**

Two major meridians, energetic pathways (transport jing, chi) ⇨ up spine, front, back ⇨ head, mouth
- Du ⇨ back, feeds yang organs: GB, UB, LI, SI, ST
- Ren ⇨ up, feeds yin organs: LV, K, SP, HT, LG

1. Close eyes. Breathe deeply one minute. Touch the tongue to roof of mouth (unites Du, Ren)

2. **Inhale** breath ⇨ nose ⇩ lungs ⇩ lower abdomen ⇩ perineum (midway scrotum, vagina, anus), hold 5 sec. ⇨ **Du** up ⇧ back, along spine ⇧ back ⇧ neck ⇧ head ⇩ middle forehead ⇩ nose ⇩ mouth (roof)

3. **Exhale** down ⇩ throat ⇩ **Ren**, front ⇩ middle of chest ⇩ abdomen ⇩ perineum. Relax few seconds.

4. Repeat 20+ minutes, relax ⇨ increases benefit, circulation of energy

This meditation circulates energy around, energizes the brain, spine as well as the chakras. My experience, spine became a hollow tunnel in which I could hear, feel a hollow, windy sound (sea shell).

III. Spiritual meditations
- Generally, focus on God, move, concentrate energy, thought within or around (like Du, Ren) the brain, spine, chakras.
- Require purity, health, patience and guidance from experienced practitioners, as incorrect practice or an increase in spiritual energy can easily damage, burn an unhealthy, unprepared nervous system, just as excessive electrical voltage can easily shatter a lamp-bulb

I (beginner) practice Kriya Yoga, spiritual meditation (Self-Realization Fellowship, CA). My general experience is a feeling of peace, joy, love and sometimes more.

"Spiritual truth and wisdom are found not in the words of a priest or preacher, but in the "wilderness" of inner silence." page 122. "Seclusion is the price of greatness and God-contact." Paramahansa Yogananda, **The Second Coming of Jesus Christ**, page 258.

Section IV. Appendices

ABOUT THE AUTHOR

1955 (age 3), while sitting outdoors, sun shining and putting on band aid, I had a vision, I would be a doctor, although the only doctor I knew and disliked (needles, pain) was an M.D. (needle pain). The doctor I eventually became, Acupuncture Physician (L.Ac.) specializing more in Ayurvedic medicine, diet, herbs, exercise than Chinese medicine and needles; as well as owner of a small health food store and author, was far different, unexpected.

By my early twenties, I was convinced via intuition that maintaining health and curing most disease did not for the most part require doctors, drugs, etc., but instead good education, diet, exercise, positivity, patience, and the ability to suffer some pain, which is how I really learned (later on, questioning, counseling many) biology, diagnosis, natural healing, food, herbal medicine, etc.

I have never carried health insurance, until age 65, free Medicare Part A (unused). The dentist is another story $$$. Sugar. Last **45 years**: $600 on five doctors: strep throat (1978), three water on knee (basketball, 50's), general exam (2008), no colds, flus, flu shot, have suffered and cured many diseases, caused by poor diet. I have not always eaten well.

1962 (10): mother (42): breast cancer: radical mastectomy (entire breast, surrounding tissues), numerous visits, doctors, chemotherapy, radiation. I accompanied my mom and dad many times to the hospital, sat in radiation ward, watched her, others wheeled in, out via platted glass rooms, always worse, devastated, look of horror. My mom suffered greatly: disfigurement, chest: burnt skin, 5" scar, wound (always bled), edema (elephant arms, 3x swollen), insomnia, depression, yet the doctors were always willing to medicate, operate, radiate, whatever the risk, pain, suffering, death. She passed 17 years later (59).

1971 University of Pittsburgh ⇨ pre-med program. Two years later ⇨ disillusioned with organic chemistry, microbiology, calculus, little or no diet, nutrition ⇨ switched majors (political science, lawyer), started reading books: diet, nutrition, herbs, yoga, etc.

1973 shopping, working at Semple Street Food Coop, Oakland, suburb of Pittsburgh. I read **Be Here Now** by Ram Dass (Dr. Richard Alpert, Harvard, colleague of Dr. Timothy Leary), told his story, transformation from Western Psychology to Hinduism. I did not understand most of the book, except for diet and yoga. I started practicing yoga and was surprised at how calm, relaxed, flexible I felt, became unlike basketball, football (tiring, injurious). I also changed my diet from animal flesh ⇨ **ovo** (eggs), **lacto** (dairy) **vegetarian** ⇨ **lacto** ⇨ **vegan** ⇨ **raw foods** ⇨ **fruitarian** ⇨ **sproutarian** (1978).

My **mindset** during this time: meat was bad, cancer causing and the vegetarian diet healthy, spiritual. First four years, I felt **great**, lost weight, had brighter, clearer skin, more energy, flexibility, calmness. Then I got **worse**: extreme weight loss (30 lb.), impotency, colds, flu. I was not healthy, as smart as I thought.

1977 Penn State University (nutrition, dietician), quit after six months. Not diet oriented. Head nutritionist was obese. During this time, I **fasted** (water, juice) three days. **2nd** day, painful. **3rd** felt great, more energy, clear, sharp mind. **4th** big **mistake**, broke fast: pizza ⇨ vomiting cheese, sauce, mucus, etc. ⇨ throat ⇨ mouth and nasopharynx (CH. 6), nasal cavity/ nose. I did not know to eat lightly, steamed vegetables, broth or juices before and directly after. Good lesson, lasting memory.

1978 ⇨ **Atlanta, GA** ⇨ **macrobiotic diet** via books (Michio Kushi) and classes (cooking, massage, diagnosis) by Seneca and Kay Anderson. The cooking classes were great as my previous diets while intellectually correct (food combining, raw, organic) but lousy in taste.

Now I could cook better, tastier, healthier meals ⇨ weight gain, greater energy, but was still thin.

Case history #55. Three months later (winter) I got the flu, **tonsillitis, streptococcal throat**, tried curing it naturally (diet, herbs, acupuncture). Nothing worked. **4th** day: left tonsil: completely covered with white streptococcus, **swollen 2x** its size ⇨ blocked most of my throat, could barely talk. **6th** day: hallucinating, seeing ghosts: early A.M. **8th** day ⇨ **doctor.** He asked how long? I lied, said 4 days. He gave me stern lecture (he was right) and penicillin. 20 min. later ⇨ pain, swelling, infection completely disappeared. Next day, the doctor was amazed how I had healed so quickly, that mine was the **worst** case he had ever seen, how lucky I was the tonsil did not burst, leak poisons, kill me. **Not seeing an M.D.** would have been a big, huge, deadly mistake.

1979 ⇨ **Brookline, MA** ⇨ **Kushi Institute** (study macrobiotics), worked at Erewhon (Kushi's macrobiotic wholesale company) 1 year, then administrative job (KI). I also lived in two study houses (10+ people) and received more instruction, especially cooking via Hamsa Newmark and Tonia Gagne. It was fun, great.

1981 ⇨ **Langhorne, PA** managed a small health food store and occasionally taught macrobiotics.

1982 ⇨ **Boston** ⇨ married (1983) ⇨ **North Miami Beach, FL**. macrobiotic cooking, diagnosis, shiatsu massage, weekly dinner, lecture (50+ people) in our home. I also worked full time (GM) at Unicorn Natural Foods one year before quitting to solely pursue macrobiotics.

1984- 2001 I bought small health food store (Hollywood, FL) and renamed it **Food and Thought**, as I had just finished reading a book, **Food for Thought**. I thought that diet was everything, through the perfect refrigerator, I could know God.

I questioned and counseled many of my customers (60- 80/ day, 6 days/ week), always asking, "What did you eat for breakfast, lunch and dinner, last 2 days?" Most were eating too much or too little building, cleansing, etc. I offered basic advice: **vegetarian** diet for too much building and **animal**, cooked vegetables for too little. My successes were inconsistent as my knowledge of biology, diet, herbs, etc. was limited.

1988: lecture: "Chinese medicine and Herbs" by Dan Nevel, L. Ac., inspired me ⇨ Acupressure Acupuncture Institute, Miami, FL (1989- 91), graduate ⇨ professionally licensed Acupuncture Physician (FL 1992-2002). My practice however was centered on diet, herbs and exercise, not acupuncture/ needles.

1989 I (15 years' vegetarian): eczema (CH 21). I tried every Chinese herbal remedy. None worked. I read **Ayurvedic Healing** by Dr. David Frawley, O.M.D. I leaned my diet, digestion was deficient, cold. I changed my diet: more protein, fat, cooked vegetables, **spices**, cured. This was a turning point, marked my transition from Chinese Medicine to Ayurveda and Hinduism.

1992 Licensed Acupuncture Physician trying to teach Chinese medical theory, yin, yang: difficult. A few years later, I substituted hot (yang) and cold (yin), which were easier to understand, teach, and led to **HOT AND COLD HEALTH** © 2003, original title of this book, killed 2023, listed as "no featured offers", used only by Amazon, which is why I re-issued under a new title (School of Natural Healing), ISBN.

2001- 2005 excess fat, chicken, cheese, ice cream ⇨ atherosclerosis, high blood pressure, arthritis, Plantar Fasciitis, insomnia ⇨ lacto-vegetarian, vegan ⇨ cured.

I knew how to control the body, cause and cure physical disease. What I could not control was my happiness, which was not only declining, inconsistent but also mixed with sadness, anger, etc.

Age 50, my life changed for the worse, as everything (health store, youth, basketball, sex, relationships) that once made me happy, was now gone or on the way out. I became depressed, angry and drifted for many years until one-day (2006) in NYC at a Barnes and Noble, I bought **Autobiography of a Yogi** by Paramahansa Yogananda and **Bhagavad Gita** (Hindu Bible) by Swami Kriyananda (disciple), which overwhelmed me, with not only great, easy to understand knowledge, but also great love, which I only felt via Jesus, **New Testament** (1976). The **Old Testament** did not impress (1974).

I joined Paramahansa Yogananda's Self-Realization Fellowship (Los Angeles, CA), received lessons on Hinduism, Christianity, meditation, etc. which helped me greatly. It was a new beginning that required greater discipline, refinement and patience as greater challenges would occur, especially the more disciplined I became. More bad experiences would occur and reinforce past behavior of seeing only bad and clouding or forgetting the good, which also occurred, and was the point of the story. Endure and focus only on God and doing good.

"Our merit and progress consist not in many pleasures and comforts but rather in enduring great afflictions and sufferings." Paramahansa Yogananda

Growing up I had little or no interest in religion, God. I did have three visions. (1) 10 years old at a sleep away, summer camp in a tub in a lake, sunny day when I was no longer in my bogy but just light, peace. It lasted awhile then my eyes opened and I was back in the tub. I tried to get back to that state but could not. (2) late teens I knew I would become a monk (Eastern religion, live alone), which many years later became true as my ongoing search for truth (diet, health, happiness, meaning of life) led me to seclusion, spiritual study, practice and evolution of this book from its original inception, Chinese Medicine (Taoism) to Ayurveda (Hinduism).

BIBLIOGRAPHY

1. Chang, Dr. Steven T., **The Complete System of Self-Healing, Internal Exercises**, Tao Publishing, 1985
2. Cohen, Ken, **The Way of Qigong**, Ballantine Books, 1997
3. Frantzis, B.K., **Opening the Energy Gates of Your Body**, First Atlantic N. Publishing Co., 1993

4. Frawley, Dr. David, Lad, Dr. Vasant, **Yoga of Herbs**, Lotus Press, 1986
5. Frawley, Dr. David, **Ayurvedic Healing**, Passage Press, 1989
6. **Ayurveda and the Mind**, Lotus Press, 1996
7. **Yoga and Ayurveda**, 1999
8. **Mantra Yoga and the Primal Sound**, 2010
9. **Soma Yoga**, 2012

10. Gerson, Dr. Max, M.D., **A Cancer Therapy, Results of Fifty Cases**, Totality Books, 1958
11. Green, Julian, **God's Fool, The Life and Times of Francis of Assisi**, Harper and Rowe, 1985
12. Heinerman, John, **Encyclopedia of Nuts, Berries and Seeds**, Parker Publishing Co., 1995
13. **Encyclopedia of Fruits, Vegetables, Herbs**
14. Holmes, Peter, **The Energetics of Western Herbs, Integrating Western and Oriental Herbal Medicine Traditions** (I, II), Artemis, 1989
15. Dr. Yang Jwing-Ming, **The Eight Pieces of Brocade,** Yang's Martial Arts Association, 1988
16. Kuei, Steven and Stephen Comee, **Beginning Qigong**, Charles E. Tuttle Publishing Co. Inc., 1993
17. Maciocia, Giovanni, **The Foundations of Chinese Medicine**, Churchill Livingston, 1989
18. Masahiro, Oki, **Zen Yoga Therapy**, Japan Publications Inc., 1979

19. **New Testament**

20. Ni, Hua Ching, **The Book of Changes and Unchanging Truth**, The Shrine of Eternal Breath of the Tao and College of Tao, 1983

21. Rothenberg, Dr. Mikel A., M.D. and Chapman, Charles F., **Dictionary of Medical Terms**, Barron's Educational Series, Inc. 2000

22. Tortora, Gerald J., Anagnpostakos, Nicholas P., **Principles of Anatomy and Physiology**, Harper and Row, Publishers, 1987

23. Swami Sri Yukteswar **The Holy Science** 1990

24. Paramahansa Yogananda, **Autobiography of a Yogi**, Self-Realization Fellowship (SRF), 1946

25. **Man's Eternal Quest**, SRF, 1982

26. **The Divine Romance**, SRF, 1986

27. **Journey To Self-Realization**, SRF, 1997

28. **Bhagavad-Gita**, SRF, 1995

29. **The Second Coming of Christ**, SRF, 2004

30. Swami Kriyananda (J. Donald Walters), direct disciple of Paramahansa Yogananda **Conversations with Yogananda**, 2004

31. **The Essence of the Bhagavad Gita**, 2006

32. **Revelations of Christ**, 2010

33. **Demystifying Patanjali**, 2013

34. **The Promise of Immortality**, 2001

35. Vogel, Adalbert Albert **Therese Neumann, Mystic and Stigmatist**, Clays LTD, St. Ives, 1957

36. **The Vegetarian Guide to Diet and Salad**, Walker, N.W., D. Sc., 1940

37. My apologies to the many authors not mentioned.

INDEX

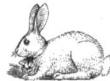

....

www.ingramcontent.com/pod-product-compliance
Lightning Source LLC
Chambersburg PA
CBHW060836280326
41934CB00007B/807